Drugs in Cancer Care

DATE DUE

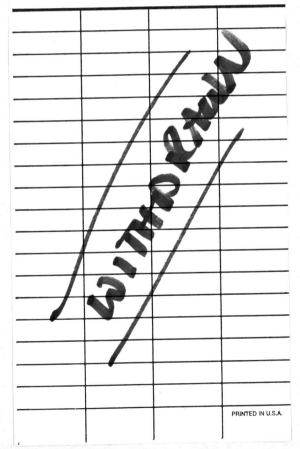

Drugs in Cancer Care

Edited by

Rachel S. Midgley

Consultant Oncologist and DH/HEFCE Clinical Senior
Lecturer
Director of the Oncology Clinical Trials Office (OCTO)
Churchill Hospital and the University of Oxford
Churchill Campus
Oxford, UK

Mark R. Middleton

Professor of Experimental Cancer Medicine and
Consultant Medical Oncologist
Department of Oncology
Oxford University Hospitals NHS Trust
Churchill Hospital
Oxford, UK

Andrew R. Dickman

Consultant Pharmacist—Palliative Care
Blackpool Teaching Hospitals NHS Foundation Trust
and Marie Curie Palliative Care Institute
Department of Molecular and Clinical Cancer Medicine
University of Liverpool, Cancer Research Centre
Liverpool, UK

David J. Kerr

Professor of Cancer Medicine
University of Oxford, UK
and Adjunct Professor of Medicine
Weill Cornell College of Medicine
New York, USA

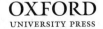

OXFORD
UNIVERSITY PRESS

OXFORD
UNIVERSITY PRESS

Great Clarendon Street, Oxford, OX2 6DP,
United Kingdom

Oxford University Press is a department of the University of Oxford.
It furthers the University's objective of excellence in research, scholarship,
and education by publishing worldwide. Oxford is a registered trade mark of
Oxford University Press in the UK and in certain other countries

ISBN 978–0–19–966457–3

Printed in Great Britain by
Ashford Colour Press Ltd, Gosport, Hampshire

Foreword

It is widely recognized that cancer care encompasses multidisciplinary delivery by surgeons, radiation and medical oncologists, supported by specialist pathologists, radiologists, pharmacists, and nurses. We have seen extraordinary advances being made at the level of cell and molecular biology which are being translated into novel targeted therapeutics, which keeps the oncology community as standard bearers for the much-promised evolution in personalized medicine. No less a person than Francis Collins, awarded the Nobel Prize for his contribution to sequencing the human genome, has declared us the medical specialty which has most fully embraced the concept of precision medicine, targeting the right drugs to the right patients at the right time in the natural history of their disease. There has never been a better time to celebrate this paradigm change in cancer medicine, whilst contextualizing it in the rich tapestry of the past, through which is woven conventional cytotoxic drugs.

Drugs in Cancer Care aims to support healthcare professionals, including doctors, nurses, and pharmacists involved in the management of cancer patients, by providing pertinent information in an easily accessible format about many of the medicines likely to be encountered in their management, both with curative and palliative intent. This edition offers up-to-date information presented in a logical and comprehensive way, from basic clinical pharmacology through to succinct monographs. There is clear indexing to enable readers to access specific drugs and cross-referencing to other relevant areas.

This book has a place in everyday practice in cancer care, both for the specialist and also the generalist in supporting decision-making and prescribing for cancer patients. It will enable the healthcare professional to make the most appropriate choice of drug at the right dose for the right disease, the right stage, and the right symptom. Good cancer care is only as good as the multidisciplinary healthcare professionals providing it. This book will function as an essential cornucopia of immensely practical information that will contribute to improving quality and reducing harm.

David J. Kerr CBE MA MD DSc FRCP FRCGP FMedSci
Professor of Cancer Medicine, University of Oxford
Adjunct Professor of Medicine, Weill Cornell College
of Medicine, New York
President of European Society of Medical Oncology, 2009–2011

Foreword

Contents

Detailed Contents

Acknowledgements

Chapter 1 'Clinical pharmacology overview' has been adapted from Andrew Dickman, *Drugs in Palliative Care, Second Edition*, Oxford University Press, Copyright © Andrew Dickman 2012, with permission of Oxford University Press.

The following vignettes have been reproduced from Andrew Dickman, *Drugs in Palliative Care, Second Edition*, Oxford University Press, Copyright © Andrew Dickman 2012, with permission of Oxford University Press.

- Anastrozole
- Cyproterone
- Diethylstilboestrol
- Erlotinib
- Exemestane
- Imatanib
- Letrozole
- Medroxyprogesterone acetate
- Megestrol acetate
- Melphalan
- Tamoxifen
- Thalidomide.

Contributors

David Church
Medical Oncology Registrar
The Churchill Hospital
Oxford University Hospitals
NHS Trust
Oxford, UK

Graham Collins
Consultant Haematologist
The Churchill Hospital
Oxford University Hospitals
NHS Trust
Oxford, UK

Avinash Gupta
Medical Oncology Registrar
The Churchill Hospital
Oxford University Hospitals
NHS Trust
Oxford, UK

Nicola Levitt
Consultant in Medical Oncology
The Churchill Hospital
Oxford University Hospitals
NHS Trust
Oxford, UK

Shibani Nicum
Consultant in Medical Oncology
The Churchill Hospital
Oxford University Hospitals
NHS Trust
Oxford, UK

Andrew Protheroe
Consultant in Medical Oncology
The Churchill Hospital
Oxford University Hospitals
NHS Trust
Oxford, UK

Symbols and Abbreviations

📖	cross-reference
🜪	dose/dose adjustments
⊕	pharmacology
☺	undesirable effects
¥	unlicensed indication
❶	warning
↑	increased
↓	decreased
~	approximately
5FU	fluorouracil
5-HT	serotonin
ACE	angiotensin-converting enzyme
ACTH	adrenocorticotropic hormone
ADCC	antibody-dependent cellular cytotoxicity
AIDS	acquired immune deficiency syndrome
ALT	alanine aminotransferase
AML	acute myeloid leukaemia
ANC	absolute neutrophil count
APTT	activated partial thromboplastin time
AST	aspartate aminotransferase
AUC	area under the concentration–time curve
BCG	Bacillus Calmette–Guérin
BD	*bis die* (twice a day)
BSA	body surface area
CHF	congestive heart failure
CLL	chronic lymphocytic leukaemia
CML	chronic myeloid leukaemia
CMV	cytomegalovirus
CNS	central nervous system
CrCl	creatinine clearance
CSF	cerebrospinal fluid
cuSCC	cutaneous squamous cell carcinoma
DHEA	dehydroepiandrosterone
DHFR	dihydrofolate reductase
DNA	deoxyribonucleic acid
DVT	deep vein thrombosis
ECG	electrocardiogram

ECOG	Eastern Cooperative Oncology Group
EGF	epidermal growth factor
EGFR	epidermal growth factor receptor
eGFR	estimated glomerular filtration rate
FSH	follicle stimulating hormone
G6PD	glucose-6-phosphate dehydrogenase
GFR	glomerular filtration rate
GFRABS	absolute glomerular filtration rate
GI	gastrointestinal
GIST	gastrointestinal stromal tumour
GnRH	gonadotropin-releasing hormone
GTD	gestational trophoblastic disease
HDAC	histone deacetylase
HER	human epidermal growth factor receptor
HIV	human immunodeficiency virus
HNSCC	head and neck squamous cell carcinoma
HPCT	haematopoietic progenitor cell transplantation
Ig	immunoglobulin
IL	interleukin
IM	intramuscular
INR	international normalized ratio
IU	international unit
IV	intravenous
K$^+$	potassium
LFT	liver function test
LH	luteinizing hormone
LHRH	luteinizing hormone-releasing hormone
LVEF	left ventricular ejection fraction
MAO	monoamine oxidase
MDS	myelodysplastic syndrome
MIU	million international units
MTIC	methyl triazenoimidazole carboxamide
mTOR	mammalian target of rapamycin
NK	natural killer
NRI	noradrenaline reuptake inhibitor
NSAID	non-steroidal anti-inflammatory drug
NSCLC	non-small cell lung cancer
NSGCT	non-seminoma germ cell tumour
OD	*omni die* (once a day)
ONJ	osteonecrosis of the jaw
PCR	polymerase chain reaction

PE	pulmonary embolus
P-gp	P-glycoprotein
PM	poor metabolizer
PO	*per os* (by mouth)
POM	prescription-only medicine
PPE	palmar–plantar erythrodysaesthesia
PPI	proton pump inhibitor
PT	prothrombin time
QDS	*quater die sumendus* (four times daily)
RNA	ribonucleic acid
RPLS	reversible posterior leucoencephalopathy syndrome
SC	subcutaneous
SIADH	syndrome of inappropriate antidiuretic hormone secretion
SNP	single nucleotide polymorphism
SPC	Summary of Product Characteristics
SSRI	selective serotonin reuptake inhibitor
STS	soft tissue sarcoma
TDS	*ter die sumendus* (three times daily)
TNM	tumour, node, metastasis
TPMT	thiopurine methyltransferase
TS	thymidylate synthase
ULN	upper limit of normal
UM	ultrarapid metabolizer
VEGF	vascular endothelial growth factor
VEGFR	vascular endothelial growth factor receptor
VTE	venous thromboembolism
WBC	white blood cell

Clinical pharmacology overview

Rationale for combination cancer therapy

When any drugs are administered in combination, 3 outcomes are possible, namely: additive effects—the drugs act completely independently of each other, presumably through non-overlapping biochemical pathways, and have no pharmacokinetic interactions which alter the quantum of drug reaching its active site; subtractive or negative synergistic effects—whereby one drug interferes with the other to reduce efficacy. This could be competition at the active site, altered pharmacokinetics, say by inducing one of the enzyme systems responsible for the other drug's metabolism, or the unexpected consequence that inhibition of a biochemical pathway might have on up/downregulation of the target of the companion drug. Synergy is defined as an interaction between drugs where the effects are stronger than their mere sum and may be driven by both pharmacokinetic and pharmacodynamic interactions. Probably the best way of demonstrating true synergy is to use the Chou–Talalay method for drug combination which is based on the median-effect equation, derived from the mass-action law principle. This is the unified theory that provides the common link between single entity and multiple entities, and first-order and higher-order dynamics. It is possible, therefore, to apply stringent equations in the preclinical setting, both *in vitro* and *in vivo*, to empirical cytotoxic drug combinations to determine whether true synergy can be documented and therefore used as supporting evidence to take specific anticancer drug combinations through into the clinic.

At a more prosaic level, the early guiding principles for selecting cytotoxic drug combinations were very simple: drugs which had some level of single-agent activity for particular tumour types; a distinct mechanism of action, as it was thought that this might eliminate or at least delay the outgrowth of drug-resistant clones; as far as possible, non-overlapping toxicity, the overall aim being to administer both drugs at as close to their single-agent doses as was tolerable. This was packaged mathematically by some rational equations of the day (Goldie–Coldman, Norton–Day) which focused on chemotherapy resistance. Needless to say, the rather empirical preclinical models were not hugely predictive of clinical synergy.

We are now entering the new age of mechanism-oriented rational prediction of synergy. There are bioinformaticians who are attempting to understand the consequences that perturbing a specific biochemical pathway with drug X will have on other related cellular functions. This implies sufficient knowledge of the interconnectedness of cell signalling, crosstalk between pathways, and inherent redundancy, all of which add up to a complex system that requires significant computing power and mathematical modelling to resolve. Although this field is in its relative infancy, advances are being made, fuelled by the increasing availability of sophisticated genomic tools (next-generation sequencing, single-nucleotide polymorphism (SNP) typing, polymerase chain reaction (PCR)) and the willingness of cancer patients and their oncologists to consider biopsy of disease on progression of first-line therapy.

For example, the drug crizotinib was approved for use with the subset of non-small cell lung cancer (NSCLC) patients with chromosomal rearrangements involving the anaplastic lymphoma kinase (*ALK*) gene, or simply 'ALK-positive' patients. Unfortunately (as with many drugs), ALK+ NSCLC tends to develop resistance to crizotinib. Multiple resistance mutations in the *ALK* gene, often affecting the conformation of its active site, have now been described by sequencing the gene in patients with progressive cancer; however, there are new data to suggest that when *ALK* is targeted, human tumours can switch their dependence, or oncogene addiction, from ALK to either *KRAS* or epidermal growth factor receptor (*EGFR*) mutations. One would predict that initial combinations of ALK and EGFR inhibitors would be a logical way of overcoming, preventing, or delaying the emergence of resistant disease. Thus providing a molecular rationale for a drug combination which meets our old criteria—drugs with single-agent activity for NSCLC, different spectra of toxicity, and unique modes of action. It is gratifying that some of the early principles of cancer therapy are sufficiently flexible to adapt to the molecular age!

Anticancer drug taxonomies

Introduction

It is interesting to reflect that the first seekers of knowledge sought to classify, to explain the known universe through taxonomy. Little has changed in the ensuing millennia. Oncologists are no different in this regard, grouping cancers by organ of origin, by TNM (tumour, node, metastasis) stage, and increasingly, biomarkers which may be used for prognostic or predictive purposes—welcome to the age in which cancer is being increasingly referred to as a group of a 'thousand rare diseases, each defined by clustered genotype'.

This is true too of our desire to clump different drug classes together, although on reflection, this could be done in many different ways—most commonly, shared elements of chemical structure (the anthracyclines, vinca alkaloids, taxanes, fluoropyrimidines) and/or mechanism of action (the alkylating agents, EGFR inhibitors, ALK inhibitors, mammalian target of rapamycin (mTOR) inhibitors, multitargeted kinase inhibitors, etc.). It is less usual to see drugs classified broadly into disease-specific families, e.g. colorectal cancer: 5-fluorouracil (5-FU), capecitabine, S1, UFT, oxaliplatin, irinotecan, mitomycin, bevacizumab, cetuximab, regorafenib, aflibercept, or according to toxicity, e.g. peripheral neurotoxicity: cisplatin, oxaliplatin, carboplatin, vincristine, vinblastine, paclitaxel, docetaxel, suramin, thalidomide. The latter taxonomies are likely to be more clinically useful to the general oncologist in terms of pointing towards likely candidates for specific tumours and the ensuing pattern of toxicity, but as we embrace a more target-oriented approach to cancer therapy, one would hope that the dominant descriptive categories are related to mechanisms of action.

DNA synthesis inhibitors

Anthracyclines (Adriamycin®, daunomycin, epirubicin, daunorubicin)

Are a class of antitumour antibiotics used in cancer chemotherapy derived from the *Streptomyces* bacteria and have 3 mechanisms of action:

- Inhibits DNA and RNA synthesis by intercalating between base pairs of the DNA/RNA strand, thus preventing the replication of rapidly-growing cancer cells.
- Inhibits topoisomerase II enzyme, preventing the relaxing of supercoiled DNA and thus blocking DNA transcription and replication.
- Creates iron-mediated free oxygen radicals that damage the DNA and the lipid domain of cell membranes.

Vinca alkaloids (vincristine, vinorelbine, vinblastine, vindesine)

Are a set of antimitotic and antimicrotubule agents that were originally derived from the periwinkle plant *Catharanthus roseus*. The principal mechanisms of cytotoxicity relate to their interactions with tubulin and disruption of microtubule function, particularly of microtubules comprising the mitotic spindle apparatus, leading to metaphase arrest.

Taxanes (docetaxel, paclitaxel)

Taxanes are diterpenes produced by plants of the genus *Taxus* (yews). The principal mechanism of action of the taxane class of drugs is the disruption of microtubule function. Microtubules are essential to cell division, and taxanes stabilize guanosine diphosphate (GDP)-bound tubulin in the microtubule, thereby inhibiting the process of cell division—a 'frozen mitosis'. Thus, in essence, taxanes are mitotic inhibitors. In contrast to the taxanes, the vinca alkaloids destroy mitotic spindles. Both taxanes and vinca alkaloids are, therefore, named spindle poisons.

Alkylating agents (nitrogen mustards—cyclophosphamide, ifosfamide, melphalan, chlorambucil; nitrosoureas—carmustine, lomustine, streptozotocin; alkyl sulphonate—busulfan)

Their principal mechanism of action is to alkylate the N7 residue of the guanine which can crosslink nucleobases in DNA double-helix strands. This makes the strands unable to uncoil and separate leading ultimately to apoptotic cell death. The antitumour antibiotic, mitomycin isolated from *Streptomyces caespitosus*, can also be considered an alkylating agent as it is activated to produce a species which crosslinks guanine residues in the sequence 5'-CpG-3'.

Bleomycin

Is a glycopeptide antibiotic produced by the bacterium *Streptomyces verticillus* which induces DNA strand breaks by generating superoxide free radicals.

Platinum-based agents (cisplatin, carboplatin, oxaliplatin)

Platinum-based agents also bind N7 guanine and can cause intra- and interstrand DNA crosslinks, inhibiting DNA synthesis and inducing programmed cell death.

Antimetabolites (purines, pyrimidines, antifolates)

An antimetabolite is a chemical that inhibits the use of a naturally occurring metabolite, which is essential for the cell's normal economy, e.g. DNA and protein synthesis. Such drugs are often similar in structure to the metabolite with which they interfere.

Purine analogues (mercaptopurine, thioguanine, fludarabine, pentostatin and cladribine)

Are antimetabolites that mimic the structure of metabolic purines and which therefore inhibit DNA synthesis.

Pyrimidine analogues (5-FU, gemcitabine, floxuridine, cytosine arabinoside)

Are antimetabolites which mimic the structure of metabolic pyrimidines and which inhibit DNA and RNA synthesis.

Antifolate analogues (methotrexate, pemetrexed)

Are drugs that impair the function of folic acids. A well-known example is methotrexate. This is a folic acid analogue, and owing to structural similarity with it binds and inhibits the enzyme dihydrofolate reductase (DHFR), and thus prevents the formation of tetrahydrofolate. Because tetrahydrofolate is essential for purine and pyrimidine synthesis, methotrexate inhibits production of DNA, RNA, and proteins (as tetrahydrofolate is also involved in the synthesis of amino acids serine and methionine).

Topoisomerase inhibitors (topo 1—irinotecan, topotecan;
topo 2—etoposide, amsacrine, teniposide)
Inhibit the 2 enzymes that regulate the overwinding or underwinding of
DNA and lead to single- and double-strand DNA breaks that can induce
apoptosis.

Hormonal agents

Hormonal therapy involves the manipulation of the endocrine system
through exogenous administration of specific hormones, particularly steroid hormones, or drugs which inhibit the production or activity of such
hormones (hormone antagonists). Because steroid hormones are power-
ful drivers of gene expression in certain cancer cells, changing the levels or
activity of certain hormones can cause cytostasis, or cell death.

Inhibitors of hormone synthesis
Aromatase inhibitors
At menopause, oestrogen production in the ovaries ceases, but other tissues continue to produce oestrogen through the action of the enzyme
aromatase on androgens produced by the adrenal glands. Aromatase
blockade reduces oestrogen levels in postmenopausal women, causing growth arrest and/or apoptosis of hormone-responsive cancer cells.
Letrozole and anastrozole are aromatase inhibitors which have been
shown to be superior to tamoxifen for the first-line treatment of breast
cancer in postmenopausal women and exemestane is an irreversible
'aromatase inactivator' which is superior to megestrol for treatment of
tamoxifen-refractory metastatic breast cancer.

Gonadotropin-releasing hormone (GnRH) analogues
Analogues of GnRH can induce chemical castration, and complete suppression of the production of oestrogen, progesterone, and testosterone
from the reproductive organs via the negative feedback effect of continuous stimulation of the pituitary gland by these hormones. Leuprolide and
goserelin are GnRH analogues that are used primarily for the treatment of
hormone-responsive prostate cancer.

Selective oestrogen receptor modulators (SERMs)
Tamoxifen is a partial agonist, which can actually increase oestrogen
receptor signalling in some tissues, such as the endometrium. Raloxifene is
another partial agonist SERM which does not seem to promote endometrial cancer, and is used primarily for chemoprevention of breast cancer
in high-risk individuals. Toremifene and fulvestrant are SERMs with little
or no agonist activity.

Antiandrogens (flutamide, bicalutamide)
Antiandrogens are a class of drug which bind and inhibit the androgen
receptor, blocking the growth- and survival-promoting effects of testosterone on certain prostate cancers.

Cell signalling inhibitors
This broad classification underpins the remarkable insights that cell and
molecular biology have yielded over the past 2 decades that have resulted

in drugable targets, several of which are used as biomarkers to select chemosensitive patient subpopulations.

Angiogenesis inhibitors (bevacizumab, aflibercept, sorafenib, sunitinib, pazopanib, and everolimus)

Angiogenesis requires the binding of signalling molecules, such as vascular endothelial growth factor (VEGF), to receptors on the surface of normal endothelial cells. When VEGF and other endothelial growth factors bind to their receptors on endothelial cells, signals within these cells are initiated that promote the growth and survival of new blood vessels.

Angiogenesis inhibitors interfere with various steps in this process, e.g. bevacizumab is a monoclonal antibody that specifically recognizes and binds to VEGF, preventing it from activating its receptor. Other angiogenesis inhibitors, including sorafenib and sunitinib, bind to receptors on the surface of endothelial cells or to other proteins in the downstream signalling pathways, blocking their activities.

Growth factor receptor inhibitors

Aberrant expression of the EGFR system has been reported in a wide range of epithelial cancers. In some studies, this has also been associated with a poor prognosis and resistance to the conventional forms of therapies. These discoveries have led to the strategic development of several kinds of EGFR inhibitors, five of which have gained US Food and Drug Administration approval for the treatment of patients with NSCLC (gefitinib and erlotinib), metastatic colorectal cancer (cetuximab and panitumumab), head and neck cancer (cetuximab), pancreatic cancer (erlotinib), and breast cancer (lapatinib). These comprise the anti-EGFR monoclonal antibodies cetuximab and panitumumab and the small molecule EGFR tyrosine kinase inhibitors gefitinib and erlotinib. Human epidermal growth factor receptor 2 (HER2) is the target of the monoclonal antibody, trastuzumab, which is effective only in cancers where HER2 is overexpressed.

One of the difficulties in classifying signal transduction inhibitors is that they often have multiple targets and it may be impossible to be precise about the dominant mode of action. Some of the main pharmacological types are:

- Tyrosine kinase inhibitors:
  - These include erlotinib, imatinib, gefitinib, dasatinib, sunitinib, nilotinib, lapatinib, sorafenib, crizotinib, trametinib, vemurafenib.
- Proteasome inhibitors:
  - Bortezomib.
- mTOR inhibitors:
  - Temsirolimus, everolimus.
- Histone deacetylase inhibitors (HDACs):
  - HDACs used in cancer treatment or in clinical trials include vorinostat (suberoylanilide hydroxamic acid, SAHA), belinostat, panobinostat, entinostat and mocetinostat.
- Hedgehog pathway inhibitors:
  - Vismodegib.

Pharmacokinetics

The rate and manner that a drug is absorbed, distributed, metabolised and eliminated is described by pharmacokinetics. In other words, *what the body does to the drug*.

Absorption

The bioavailability of a drug describes the proportion of a dose of a drug that enters the systemic circulation, e.g. for intravenous (IV) morphine this would be 100% compared to 15–65% for oral morphine.

For drugs taken orally that are intended for systemic action, a significant proportion of a given dose may not even enter the systemic circulation. This may be due to poor absorption from the gastrointestinal (GI) tract, or metabolism in the gut wall or liver (called first-pass metabolism—see Box 1.1).

Box 1.1 First-pass metabolism

First-pass metabolism is a term used to describe the metabolism that occurs between the gut lumen and the systemic circulation. It can reduce the bioavailability of a drug so much so that oral administration is not feasible. Although gastric secretions inactivate certain drugs (e.g. insulin), the main sites of first-pass metabolism are the gut wall and liver.

The cytochrome P450 isoenzyme CYP3A4 (see 📖 Box 1.3, p.11) is located in the gut wall and liver. It metabolizes many drugs and therefore alterations in CYP3A4 activity can significantly influence bioavailability. It is susceptible to inhibition and induction by a variety of drugs and foods. For example, one glass of grapefruit juice can cause significant inhibition of intestinal CYP3A4 while repeated consumption can interfere with hepatic CYP3A4. The majority of orally administered drugs must pass through the liver before entering the systemic circulation. Some drugs are susceptible to extensive first-pass metabolism such that only a small proportion of the oral dose enters the systemic circulation, which renders oral administration impossible (e.g. lidocaine, fentanyl).

First-pass metabolism can be affected by disease, genetic influences, and enzyme inhibition or induction. This helps to explain the wide inter-patient variation in drug absorption and hence bioavailability of several drugs (e.g. morphine 15–65%).

Several transporter proteins are present in the intestines which influence the absorption of drugs. P-glycoprotein (P-gp) is an efflux transporter molecule that can affect the bioavailability and intracellular concentrations of several cytotoxic agents (see Box 1.2). Less well-categorized influx transporter proteins are also present and their activity may well be influenced by drugs and food.

Box 1.2 The P-gp drug transporter

P-gp is one of many protein transporters that can influence the bioavail-ability, distribution, and elimination of many drugs relevant to oncology, e.g. P-gp is believed to be a major determinant of the bioavailability of morphine and tramadol. It is found in the GI tract, kidney, liver, and blood–brain barrier. There is wide patient variation because P-gp is genetically encoded and is subject to polymorphism. Drug interactions can occur through induction or inhibition of P-gp, the clinical significance of which are just being realized. At the level of the cancer cell, P-gp functions as a drug efflux pump and can contribute to resistance against anthracyclines, taxanes, vinca alkaloids, etoposide, and mitomycin.

Distribution

Many drugs, such as albumin, bind to plasma proteins. Bound drug is inac-tive; only unbound drug is available to bind to receptors or to cross cell membranes.

Changes in protein binding can alter a drug's distribution, although this is rarely clinically important (with the exception of phenytoin).

P-gp is involved in the distribution of several drugs across the blood–brain barrier, e.g. P-gp limits the entry of morphine into the brain.

Elimination

Various processes are involved in drug elimination, although hepatic and renal processes are the most important.

Metabolism

The liver is the main organ of drug metabolism. There are generally 2 types of reaction (Phase I and Phase II) that have 2 important effects:
• To make the drug more water soluble—to aid excretion by the kidneys.
• To inactivate the drug—in most cases the metabolite is less active than the parent drug, although in some cases the metabolite can be as active, or more so, than the parent. Prodrugs are inactive until metabolized to the active drug (e.g. irinotecan is a water-soluble prodrug of the active metabolite SN38).

Phase I metabolism involves oxidation, reduction, or hydrolysis reactions. Oxidation reactions are most common and are catalysed by cytochrome P450 isoenzymes (see Box 1.3) located primarily in the liver. The main exception is CYP3A4, which is also located in the GI tract.

Phase II metabolism involves conjugation reactions, such as glucuronida-tion or sulphation, which produce more water-soluble compounds, ena-bling rapid elimination.

Many drugs are dependent on cytochrome P450 isoenzymes for metab-olism and/or elimination. Genetic variations or co-administration of induc-ers or inhibitors can lead to the development of significant toxicity or lack of effect.

Drug excretion

The main route of excretion of drugs is the kidney. Renal elimination is dependent on multiple factors that include:

- Glomerular filtration rate (GFR).
- Active tubular secretion (may involve P-gp).
- Passive tubular secretion.

If a drug is metabolized to mainly inactive compounds (e.g. 5-FU), renal function will not greatly affect the elimination. If, however, the drug is excreted largely unchanged (e.g. carboplatin), or an active metabolite is excreted via the kidney (e.g. morphine), changes in renal function will influence the elimination. Dose adjustments may be necessary.

Box 1.3 The cytochrome P450 system C1.B5

The cytochrome P450 system consists of a large group of >500 isoenzymes that are involved in the metabolism of endogenous (e.g. steroids, eicosanoids) and exogenous (e.g. drugs) compounds. They are grouped according to amino acid sequence; a family is defined by >40% homology and a subfamily is defined by >55% homology. Five subfamilies, CYP1A, CYP2C, CYP2D, CYP2E, and CYP3A, have a major role in hepatic drug metabolism, with others having a lesser role. The following list briefly describes the isoenzymes involved.

CYP1A subfamily

- CYP1A1: mainly found in lungs and metabolizes tobacco to potentially carcinogenic substances.
- CYP1A2: responsible for metabolism of ~15% of drugs; is induced by tobacco smoke. Also involved in activation of procarcinogens. Polymorphisms exist, but distribution remains undetermined. Important substrates include flutamide, olanzapine, and theophylline.

CYP2A subfamily

- CYP2A6: metabolizes a small number of drugs including nicotine and the prodrug tegafur. Also metabolizes tobacco to potentially carcinogenic substances. Polymorphisms exist, with 1% of the Caucasian population being poor metabolizers (PMs).

CYP2B subfamily

- CYP2B6: involved in the metabolism of an increasing number of drugs including cyclophosphamide and ifosfamide. Clopidogrel is a potentially potent inhibitor, while rifampicin induces this isoenzyme. Polymorphisms exist, but distribution and consequence remain undetermined.

CYP2C subfamily

- CYP2C8: a major hepatic cytochrome and shares substrates with CYP2C9 and is involved in metabolism of paclitaxel. Polymorphisms exist, but distribution and consequence remain undetermined.
- CYP2C9: the most important of the CYP2C subfamily. Responsible for the metabolism of many drugs, including tamoxifen, warfarin, celecoxib, ibuprofen, diclofenac, and phenytoin. Is inhibited by

Box 1.3 (Cont'd)

several drugs including fluconazole; rifampicin induces activity of CYP2C9. Polymorphisms exist; 1–3% of Caucasians have reduced activity and are PMs.

- CYP2C19: involved in the metabolism of several drugs, including tamoxifen, omeprazole, lansoprazole, diazepam, and citalopram. Inhibitors include modafinil, omeprazole, and fluoxetine. Carbamazepine can induce this isoenzyme. 3–5% of Caucasians lack the enzyme and are PMs.

CYP2D subfamily

- CYP2D6: no known inducer. Responsible for the metabolism of >25% of drugs, including codeine, tramadol, and tamoxifen. 5–10% of Caucasians lack this enzyme and are termed PMs; 1–5% have multiple copies of the gene and are termed ultrarapid metabolizers (UMs).

CYP2E subfamily

- CYP2E1: has a minor role in drug metabolism. Main importance is paracetamol metabolism and potential toxicity. Polymorphisms exist, but distribution and consequence remain undetermined.

CYP3A subfamily

This subfamily is the most abundant in the liver and is responsible for the metabolism of >50% of drugs, including docetaxel, exemestane, gefitinib, teniposide, vinblastine, vincristine, and ifosfamide. There are 4 *CYP3A* genes, although only 2 are likely to be of importance in human adults. Nonetheless, these isoenzymes are so closely related that they are often referred to collectively as CYP3A. Polymorphisms exist, but distribution and consequence remain undetermined.

- CYP3A4: most significant isoenzyme involved in drug metabolism and is frequently implicated in drug interactions (cyclophosphamide, etoposide). It is located mainly in the liver, but significant amounts are present in the GI tract, where it has an important role in first-pass metabolism. There are several inducers (e.g. carbamazepine, rifampicin) and inhibitors (e.g. clarithromycin, grapefruit juice).
- CYP3A5: similar substrate spectrum to CYP3A4, but is possibly less efficient, so is unlikely to have such a dramatic effect on drug metabolism.

Pharmacodynamics

The effect of the drug and how it works in terms of its interaction with a receptor or site of action is described by pharmacodynamics. In other words, what the drug does to the body.

Most drugs act upon proteins:

- Receptor (e.g. tamoxifen and the oestrogen receptor).
- Enzyme (e.g. methotrexate's inhibition of dihydrofolate reductase).
- Transporter complex (e.g. P-gp as a drug target).
- Several cytotoxic drugs act directly on DNA:
  - Alkylating and platinating agents transfer alkyl or platinum complexes on to N7 guanine residues causing inter- and intrastrand DNA crosslinks.
  - The antitumour antibiotic bleomycin produces DNA strand breaks by free radical production.
  - Anthracyclines intercalate into the minor groove of DNA, inhibiting DNA synthesis.

The term 'receptor' is used loosely to describe the earlier listed protein targets:

- *Agonists* bind to and activate receptors to produce an effect.
- *Antagonists* also bind to receptors, without causing activation. They may prevent the action of, or displace, an agonist.
- *Partial agonists* activate receptors to a limited extent, but may also interfere with the action of the full agonist. The circumstances in which a partial agonist may act as an antagonist or an agonist depends on both the efficacy (see later in list) of the drug and the pre-existing state of receptor occupation by an agonist, e.g. buprenorphine will generally act as an antagonist if a patient is using excessive doses of morphine. At lower doses of morphine, buprenorphine will act as an agonist.
- *Affinity* is a term used to describe the tendency of a drug to bind to its receptors, e.g. naloxone has higher affinity for opioid receptors than morphine, hence its use in opioid toxicity.
- The *intrinsic activity* of a drug describes its ability to elicit an effect.
- *Efficacy* refers to the potential maximum activation of a receptor and therefore desired response, i.e. a full agonist has high efficacy, a partial agonist has medium efficacy, and an antagonist has zero efficacy.
- *Potency* refers to the amount of drug necessary to produce an effect, e.g. fentanyl is more potent than morphine since the same analgesic effect occurs at much lower doses (micrograms vs. milligrams).
- Very few drugs are specific for a particular receptor or site of action and most display a degree of relative selectivity. Selectivity refers to the degree by which a drug binds to a receptor relative to other receptors. In general, as doses increase, the relative selectivity reduces such that other pharmacological actions may occur, often manifesting as undesirable effects. This is particularly true of the many kinase inhibitors which were initially considered to be specific, but have later been rebranded as multi-kinase inhibitors, e.g. sorafenib.

- *Tolerance* is the decrease in therapeutic effect that may occur, over a period of time, by identical doses of a drug. Although often expected, this has yet to be conclusively identified for opioid analgesia.
- *Tachyphylaxis* is the rapid development of tolerance. It can occur with salcatonin (calcitonin), leading to a rebound hypercalcaemia.
- *Therapeutic index or margin* is the ratio between the dose producing undesired effects and the dose producing therapeutic effects. Drugs with narrow therapeutic margins are often implicated in drug interactions.
- *Competitive antagonism* describes the situation that occurs when an antagonist competes with the agonist for the binding site of receptors. In such a situation, increasing the concentration of the agonist will favour agonist binding (and vice versa). The majority of kinase inhibitors compete at the adenosine triphosphate (ATP) binding site
- *Irreversible competitive antagonism* can occur when the antagonist disassociates very slowly, or not at all, from receptors. Increasing the dose of the agonist does not reverse the situation.
- *Non-competitive antagonism* occurs when the antagonist blocks the effects of the agonist by interaction at some point other than the receptor binding site of the agonist, e.g. several inhibitors of P-gp are allosteric inhibitors.

Effect of hepatic impairment

Impaired liver function can affect the pharmacokinetics and pharmacodynamics of many anticancer drugs, e.g. anthracyclines, taxanes, vinca alkaloids, 5-FU. Reduction in hepatic blood flow and a potential fall in the number and the activity of hepatocytes can alter liver function and impact on drug clearance. Reduced synthesis of albumin can result in ↓ drug–protein binding thereby affecting the volume of distribution. Cholestasis can affect the biliary excretion of drugs and metabolites. Patients with impaired hepatic function may also develop a degree of renal impairment due to ↓ renal plasma flow and GFR. Use of the Cockcroft and Gault equation (see Box 1.4) can overestimate renal function due to a reduced synthesis of creatinine.

Unlike impaired renal function, there is no simple test that can determine the impact of liver disease on drug handling. A combination of factors needs to be considered before such impact can be assessed, which include liver function tests (LFTs), diagnosis, and physical symptoms.

In general, the metabolism of drugs is unlikely to be affected unless the patient has severe liver disease. Most problems are seen in patients with jaundice, ascites, and hepatic encephalopathy. As such, doses of drugs should be reviewed in the following situations:

- Hepatically metabolized drug with narrow therapeutic index.
- Renally excreted drug with narrow therapeutic index.
- There is a significant involvement of the cytochrome P450 system (CYP3A4/5 is highly susceptible to liver disease, while CYP2D6 appears relatively refractory).
- International normalized ratio (INR) >1.2.
- Bilirubin >100micromol/L.
- Albumin <30g/L.
- Signs of ascites and/or encephalopathy.

Where possible, dosage amendments will be discussed in each monograph in 📖 Chapter 2.

Effect of renal impairment

The elimination of several cytotoxic drugs and their metabolites is dependent upon renal function (capecitabine, carboplatin, cisplatin, methotrexate). Impaired renal function, coupled with rising urea plasma concentrations, induces changes in drug pharmacokinetics and pharmacodynamics. Implications for drug therapy include:

- ↑ risk of undesirable effects and toxicity through reduced excretion of the drug and/or metabolite(s), e.g. pregabalin, morphine.
- ↑ sensitivity to drug effects, irrespective of route of elimination, e.g. antipsychotics.
- ↑ risk of further renal impairment, e.g. non-steroidal anti-inflammatory drugs (NSAIDs).

Many of these problems can be avoided by simple adjustment of daily dose or frequency of administration. In other situations, however, an alternative drug may need to be chosen. It is worth noting that patients with end-stage renal disease may be at risk of ↑ drug toxicity due to the reduced activity of CYP3A4/5 and CYP2D6.

Estimating renal function

Unlike liver impairment, the impact of declining renal function is quantifiable. Accurate methods of determining renal function or GFR are unsuitable for routine clinical use. Serum creatinine (creatinine is a product of muscle metabolism) has been used as a simple tool to estimate GFR. However, there are serious limitations to this approach:

- As renal function deteriorates, serum creatinine increases. However, many patients may have reduced GFR but serum creatinine concentrations fall inside the conventional laboratory normal ranges, e.g. an increase from 50micromol/L to 100micromol/L is still within normal limits, even though renal function has clearly deteriorated.
- Renal function declines with age, but serum creatinine generally remains stable. Thus a 75-year-old may have the same serum creatinine as a 25-year-old, despite having a reduced renal function.

Creatinine clearance (CrCl) serves as a surrogate for GFR. It can be determined from the Cockcroft and Gault equation (see Box 1.4), which takes weight, age, gender, and serum creatinine into consideration. The majority of dosage adjustment guidelines in the monographs are based upon CrCl. There are limitations, however, with this method as it may report inaccurately for obese and underweight patients.

Box 1.4 Cockcroft and Gault equation for calculating CrCl

$\text{CrCl} = ([140 - \text{age (years)}] \times [\text{weight (kg)}] \times F)/(\text{SeCr (micromol/L)})$

Where $F = 1.23$ (♂); 1.04 (♀)

In the UK, renal function is increasingly being reported in terms of estimated GFR (eGFR), normalized to a body surface area of 1.73m². The formula used to calculate eGFR was derived from the Modification of Diet in Renal Disease (MDRD) study. eGFR assumes the patient is of average size (assumes an average body surface area of 1.73m²), allowing a figure to be determined using only serum creatinine, age, gender, and ethnic origin. It is primarily a tool for determining renal function, of which 5 categories have been described (see Table 1.1).

eGFR is only an estimate of the GFR and has not been validated for use in the following groups or clinical scenarios:
• Children (<18 years of age)
• Acute renal failure
• Pregnancy
• Oedematous states
• Muscle wasting disease states
• Amputees
• Malnourished patients.

While eGFR may be used to determine dosage adjustments in place of creatinine clearance for most drugs in patients of average build, application in cancer patients may produce erroneous results. For example, the eGFR may underestimate the degree of renal impairment in cachectic or oedematous patients resulting in excessive doses. For these patients, providing height and weight are known, it would be prudent to calculate the absolute GFR (GFR$_{ABS}$) (see Box 1.5) and use this to determine dosage adjustments.

Table 1.1 Stages of renal failure

Stage	eGFR (mL/min/1.73m2)
1 Normal GFR[a]	>90
2 Mild impairment[a]	60–89
3 Moderate impairment	30–59
4 Severe impairment	15–29
5 Established renal failure	<15

[a] The terms stage 1 and stage 2 chronic kidney disease are only applied when there are structural or functional abnormalities. If there are no such abnormalities, an eGFR ≥60 mL/min/1.73m² is regarded as normal.

Box 1.5 Calculating GFRABS and body surface area (BSA)

$$GFR_{ABS} = eGFR \times \frac{BSA}{1.73}$$

$$BSA = \sqrt{\frac{(height(cm) \times weight(kg))}{3600}}$$

Pharmacogenetics

If it were not for the great variability among individuals, medicine might as well be a science and not an art.

Sir William Osler, 1892.

Just over 50 years ago, 2 adverse drug reactions were described as being caused by genetic mechanisms. Glucose-6-phosphate dehydrogenase (G6PD) deficiency and pseudo-cholinesterase deficiency were shown to be manifestations of specific gene mutations. Two years later, in 1959, the term 'pharmacogenetics' was introduced. It was only towards the end of the last century that significant advances were made. As a result of the Human Genome Project, a broader term, 'pharmacogenomics', was introduced (see Box 1.6).

Genetic variability can affect an individual's response to drug treatment by influencing pharmacokinetic and pharmacodynamic processes, e.g. variations in genes that encode cytochrome P450 isoenzymes, drug receptors, or transport proteins can determine clinical response. Pharmacogenetics

---

Box 1.6 Basic genetic concepts

The human genome consists of 23 pairs of chromosomes (or 22 pairs of autosomes and 1 pair of sex-linked chromosomes) within which are sequences of DNA that are referred to as genes. With the exception of the sex-linked X and Y chromosomes, an individual inherits 2 copies of each gene, 1 from each parent. A gene can exist in various forms, or alleles. Only 3% of the human genome encodes proteins.

An individual's inherited genetic profile, or genotype, may be described as being:

- Homozygous dominant (i.e. a specific gene consists of 2 identical dominant alleles).
- Heterozygous (i.e. a specific gene consists of 2 different alleles, 1 usually being dominant, the other recessive).
- Homozygous recessive (i.e. a specific gene consists of 2 identical recessive alleles).

An individual's phenotype describes the observable characteristics that are a result of the genotype and environment. Particular inherited phenotypical traits may be described as being autosomal dominant or recessive.

Pharmacogenetics is the study of how variation in an individual gene affects the response to drugs which can lead to adverse drug reactions, drug toxicity, therapeutic failure, and drug interactions.

Pharmacogenomics is the study of how variation in the human genome can be used in the development of pharmaceuticals.

Polymorphisms refer to commonly occurring genetic variants (i.e. differences in DNA sequences). In most regions of the genome, a polymorphism is of little clinical consequence. However, a polymorphism in a critical coding or non-coding region can lead to altered protein synthesis or function with clinical implications such as abnormal drug responses.

can aid in the optimization of drug therapy through the identification of individuals who are likely to respond to treatment, or those who are most likely at risk of an adverse drug reaction. Although the exact proportion of adverse drug reactions caused by genetic variability is unclear, emerging evidence suggests an increasing role. Pharmacogenetic testing is currently in early development, but current examples include:

- The need for HER2 testing before initiating trastuzumab therapy.
- Crizotinib is an effective treatment for NSCLC patients whose tumours carry chromosomal translocations of the *ALK* and *ROS1* genes
- The anti-EGF monoclonal cetuximab is not effective in the 35% of colorectal cancers with mutant KRAS
- Vemurafenib is an inhibitor of mutant BRAF, used to treat melanoma

Pharmacogenetic testing has the potential to improve the safety and efficacy of several drugs commonly encountered in anticancer and palliative care, e.g. analgesics, antidepressants, and antipsychotics.

Genetic influences on pharmacokinetics

Variations in genes that encode transport proteins have been implicated in altered therapeutic response, e.g. P-gp polymorphisms have been associated with altered morphine analgesia. However, the characterization and implications of transporter protein variations are less developed when compared to drug metabolism. There is no doubt that polymorphism of metabolic enzymes has a great effect on interpatient variability.

Several polymorphisms that affect drug metabolism have been identified and there is substantial ethnic variation in distribution. Functional changes as a result of a polymorphism can have profound effects:

- Adverse drug reaction
- Toxicity
- Lack of effect
- Drug interaction.

The isoenzymes CYP2C9, CYP2C19, and CYP2D6 are responsible for >40% of cytochrome P450-mediated drug metabolism. They display high levels of polymorphism which have been shown to affect the response of individuals to many drugs (see Box 1.7). Pharmaceutical manufacturers have realized the importance of pharmacogenetics; fewer drugs will be developed that are affected by pharmacogenetic factors because potential agents will be discarded at an early stage of development.

Genetic polymorphisms of cytochrome P450 isoenzymes can be divided into 4 phenotypes:

- *Poor metabolizers* (PMs) have 2 non-functional alleles and cannot metabolize substrates.
- *Intermediate metabolizers* (IMs) have 1 non-functional allele and 1 low-activity allele, so metabolize substrates at a low rate.
- *Extensive metabolizers* (EMs) have 1 or 2 copies of a functional allele and metabolize substrates at a normal rate.
- *Ultrarapid metabolizers* (UMs) have 3 or more copies of a functional allele and metabolize substrates at an accelerated rate.

Box 1.7 Examples of the effect P450 polymorphisms have on selected drugs

- Codeine: needs to be metabolized by CYP2D6 to morphine before analgesia is observed. PMs derive no analgesia from codeine. Drugs that inhibit CYP2D6 will mimic the PM phenotype. UMs are at risk of life-threatening adverse drug reactions as codeine is metabolized at a very high rate.
- Methadone: shows complex pharmacology. Mainly metabolized by CYP3A, but CYP2B6 and CYP2D6 are also involved. PMs of CYP2B6 and CYP2D6 are at risk of developing toxicity if methadone is titrated too quickly.
- NSAIDs: there is a suggestion that specific CYP2C8/9 genotypes can cause ↑ risk of toxicity to NSAIDs.
- Tamoxifen: the active metabolite, endoxifen, is produced by a reaction involving CYP2D6. Patients with a PM phenotype are at risk of therapeutic failure with tamoxifen. Drugs that inhibit CYP2D6 will also mimic the PM phenotype and should be avoided.
- Warfarin: bleeding effects are more common with CYP2D9 polymorphisms
- Tramadol: is primarily metabolized by CYP2D6 to an active compound, M1, which is a more potent opioid agonist. PMs show a poor response to tramadol. As with codeine, drugs that inhibit CYP2D6 can mimic the PM phenotype.

The consequences of a particular phenotype depend upon the activity of the drug. PMs are at an ↑ risk of therapeutic failure (through poor metabolism to an active compound) or undesirable effects (due to excessive dose). In contrast, UMs are at ↑ risk of therapeutic failure with conventional doses due to excessive metabolism; in the case of a prodrug, rapid production of the active compound could lead to toxicity. For example, a patient with UM phenotype for CYP2D6 may rapidly convert codeine to morphine, increasing the risk of developing toxicity; a patient with PM status for CYP2D6 will derive little, if any, analgesic benefit from codeine.

Genetic influences on pharmacodynamics
Genetic polymorphisms of drug receptors, or disease-related pathways, can influence the pharmacodynamic action of drug. These are generally less well categorized than pharmacokinetic consequences. Nonetheless, genetic variations have been shown to be clinically relevant for morphine analgesia and antidepressant therapy. In the latter case, associations between serotonin transport gene polymorphisms and depression have been demonstrated. It has also been shown that genotyping for polymorphisms of certain serotonin or noradrenaline pathways can inform clinical choice of antidepressant, e.g. a patient that fails to respond to citalopram (selective serotonin reuptake inhibitor (SSRI)) could in fact respond to reboxetine (noradrenaline reuptake inhibitor (NRI)).

Drug interactions

> Be alert to the fact that all drugs taken by patients, including over-the-counter medicines, herbal products, and nutritional supplements, have the potential to cause clinically relevant drug interactions. The patient's diet can also affect drug disposition.

The pharmacological actions of a drug can be enhanced or diminished by other drugs, food, herbal products, and nutritional supplements. Clinically relevant and potentially significant drug–drug interactions are included in the monographs in 🕮 Chapter 2.

In terms of a drug–drug interaction, the actions of the object drug are altered by the precipitant in most cases. Occasionally, the actions of both object and precipitant can be affected.

While it is possible to predict the likelihood of a drug interaction, it is often difficult to predict the clinical relevance. Elderly patients or those with impaired renal and/or hepatic function are more at risk. Drug interactions may be overlooked and explained as poor compliance, or even progressive disease. Knowledge of drug interaction processes can aid in the diagnosis of unexplained or unexpected response to drug therapy.

It is impossible accurately to determine the incidence of drug interactions. Knowledge of many drug–drug interactions comes from isolated case reports and/or small studies in healthy volunteers. It is, however, possible to indirectly assess a patient's risk; there are several factors that predispose patients receiving cancer treatment to a drug interaction (see Box 1.8).

> **Box 1.8 Factors that predispose a patient to drug interactions**
> - Advancing age
> - Multiple medications
> - Compromised renal/hepatic function
> - More than one prescriber
> - Comorbidity.

While the majority of risks cannot be reduced, they can be anticipated and managed. For example, a thorough medication history should be taken upon presentation and must include over-the-counter medications, herbal products, or nutritional supplements. In some cases, changes to diet should be enquired about, e.g. the effect of warfarin can be reduced by a diet suddenly rich in leafy, green vegetables (a source of vitamin K).

As part of the multidisciplinary team, the pharmacist is an excellent source of information and is often involved in the recording of drug histories.

There are 2 main mechanisms involved in drug interactions:
- Pharmacokinetic
- Pharmacodynamic.

Pharmacokinetic

The precipitant drug alters the absorption, distribution, metabolism, or excretion of the object drug. Pharmacokinetic drug interactions are likely to be encountered in cancer care since many of the drugs used are substrates or inducers/inhibitors of cytochrome P450 isoenzymes. These interactions are often difficult to predict.

Absorption

CYP3A4, mainly found in the liver, is also present in the gut wall. It is involved in reducing the absorption of many drugs and is subject to both induction and inhibition. Grapefruit juice inhibits the action of CYP3A4 in the bowel (and liver with repeated consumption) and can lead to significant increases in bioavailability of several drugs, e.g. the bioavailability of rapamycin is increased by 350% by coingestion of grapefruit juice. This interaction can occur even after consuming just 200mL of grapefruit juice and inhibition can persist for up to 72 hours. An interaction may occur, whatever the source, e.g. fresh grapefruit and grapefruit juices including fresh, frozen, or diluted from concentrate. Drugs with a narrow therapeutic index are more likely to be affected.

The rate of absorption or amount of object drug absorbed can be altered by the precipitant. Delayed absorption is rarely of clinical relevance unless the effect of the object drug depends upon high peak plasma concentrations (e.g. the effect of paracetamol can be enhanced by combination with metoclopramide). If the amount of drug absorbed is affected, clinically relevant effects can occur.

Absorption interactions involving simple insoluble complex formation can be easily avoided by changing the administration time of the drugs involved, e.g. ciprofloxacin and antacids.

Some interactions involve the induction or inhibition of P-gp although the clinical significance of many such interactions remains unclear. Enhanced activity of P-gp will reduce the absorption and bioavailability of a drug. The effect of drugs and food on influx transporters is currently less well categorized but could well contribute to unexplained and unanticipated drug effects.

Distribution

Such interactions are usually of little clinical relevance and often involve alterations in protein binding. This can be important, in that cancer patients often have altered concentrations of serum proteins like alpha-1-acid glycoprotein that can reduce the concentration of free drug available to diffuse from the vascular compartment to its site of action.

The distribution of some drugs is dependent on the activity of P-gp, which also appears to act as a component of the blood–brain barrier, e.g. P-gp can limit the entry of hydrophilic opioids and substrate cytotoxic drugs into the brain. The clinical significance of induction or inhibition of P-gp is unclear.

Metabolism

Many drugs are metabolized via the hepatic cytochrome P450 system which is subject to both inhibition and induction.

CYP3A4 may account for up the metabolism of up to 50% of currently used drugs; CYP2D6 may account for up to 25%. The effect that smoking can have on drug therapy should not be overlooked (see Box 1.9).

Box 1.9 Smoking and potential drug interactions

- Tobacco smoke contains several polycyclic aromatic hydrocarbons (PAHs) that are potent inducers of CYP1A1, CYP1A2, and, to a lesser extent, CYP2E1. PAHs can also induce glucuronide conjugation.
- Induction of CYP1A1 in the lungs causes activation of pro-carcinogens from tobacco smoke and is believed to be a major mechanism in the development of lung cancer.
- Although CYP1A1 is not important for drug metabolism, several drugs are substrates of CYP1A2. Metabolism of these drugs can be induced by tobacco smoke, potentially resulting in increased clearance of the drug and consequent clinically significant reductions in effects. Smokers may require higher doses of these drugs.
- Note that exposure to 'second-hand' smoke can produce similar effects.
- The PAHs cause these pharmacokinetic drug interactions, not the nicotine. Thus, nicotine replacement therapy (NRT) will not cause these effects.
- Tobacco smoke and NRT are both implicated in several pharmacodynamic drug interactions. Nicotine can have an alerting effect, thereby countering the action of other drugs.
- The prescriber should consider a dosage reduction of drugs metabolized by CYP1A2 if a patient stops smoking. Similarly, doses of anxiolytics and hypnotics should be reviewed, unless NRT is initiated. If a patient starts smoking, doses of drugs metabolized by CYP1A2 may need increasing whereas doses of anxiolytics and hypnotics may need reviewing.

- Enzyme inhibition is the mechanism most often responsible for life-threatening interactions. It can also result in reduced drug effect where activation of a prodrug is required (e.g. codeine has a reduced analgesic profile when administered with CYP2D6 inhibitors). Inhibition is generally caused by competitive binding for the isoenzyme between object and precipitant. It follows that high doses of the precipitant will cause a greater degree of inhibition. Clinically relevant interactions can be evident within 2 days. The effect of enzyme inhibition generally depends upon the half-life of the precipitating drug and the therapeutic index of the object drug. The effect will decrease as blood levels fall. Note that drugs competing for the same isoenzyme can give rise to competitive inhibition. The more drugs that are co-prescribed, the greater the risk of this occurring.

- Induction can occur when the precipitant stimulates the synthesis of more isoenzyme, increasing metabolic capacity. It can take several days or even weeks to develop and may persist for a similar duration once the precipitant has been withdrawn. Problems with toxicity can occur if doses of the object drug are ↑ but are not reduced once the precipitant is stopped.
- Many drugs are not always metabolized by one specific pathway and for this reason it is often difficult precisely to predict the outcome of a drug interaction. Nonetheless, although *in vivo* data may not be available for many drugs, *in vitro* evidence of metabolism and specific cytochrome P450 isoenzyme involvement can be used to anticipate and avoid a potentially dangerous drug interaction. The drug monographs mention actual and potential drug interactions.

Elimination

In cancer care, it is likely that the most common and potentially more clinically relevant elimination drug interactions will involve renal function. For example, with advancing age, renal function declines but compensatory mechanisms are activated that involve the production of vasodilatory prostaglandins. NSAIDs can significantly impair this compensatory measure, such that there is a marked reduction in renal function and consequential risk of drug interactions with cytotoxic agents like capecitabine.

Pharmacodynamic

The pharmacological actions of the object drug are changed by the presence of the precipitant. Pharmacodynamic interactions can be additive or antagonistic in nature.

Additive

When 2 or more drugs with similar pharmacodynamic effects are co-prescribed, the additive results may result in exaggerated response or toxicity. Additive responses can occur with the main therapeutic action of the drug as well as the undesirable effects, e.g. SSRI plus tramadol may give rise to the serotonin (5-HT) syndrome (see Box 1.10).

Antagonistic

When 2 drugs with opposing pharmacodynamic effects are co-prescribed, there may be a net reduction in response to 1 or both drugs, e.g. warfarin and vitamin K, NSAIDs and angiotensin-converting enzyme (ACE) inhibitors, metoclopramide and cyclizine.

Anticancer Drug metabolism and Interactions

The CYP450 enzymes involved in anticancer drug metabolism are summarised in Box 1.10 as are relevant drug-drug interactions that can make a difference to tolerability or even efficacy of the cancer drugs.

Box 1.10 Anticancer Drug metabolism and Interactions

CYP450 subtypes and anticancer drugs

- Cyclophosphamide 2B6, 2D6 and *3A4*; Cytarabine *3A4* Docetaxel *3A4*
- Doxorubicin *3A4*; Erlotinib 1A2 and *3A4*; Etoposide *3A4* Exemestane *3A4*
- Gefitinib 2C19 and 2D6 *3A4*; Idarubicin 2D6 2C9 and 2D6; Ifosfamide *3A4*
- Imatinib mesylate* 2C9, 2D6 and *3A4*; Irinotecan *3A4*
- Ketoconazole* *3A4* and 2C9; Letrozole* 2A6 and 2C19 2A6 and *3A4*;
- Paclitaxel 2C8 and *3A4*; Tamoxifen* *3A4* 1A2, 2A6, 2B6, 2D6, 2E1 and *3A4*
- Teniposide *3A4* ; Tretinoin* 2C8 and *3A4*; Vinblastine 2D6 *3A4*
- Vincristine 2D6 *3A4* ; Vinorelbine 2D6 *3A4*

Cancer Drug Interactions

- Antacids that contain aluminium and magnesium can increase the bioavailability of capecitabine
- Antibiotics: Penicillins block the renal elimination of MTX
- Altered coagulation has been reported in patients who have taken warfarin concurrently with capecitabine
- Anticonvulsants : Carbamazepine increases systemic clearance of teniposide
- Anti-emetics : Co-administration of ondansetron withcisplatin and cyclophosphamide can result in a decrease in systemic exposure to both drugs
- Antifungal agents: Ketoconazole inhibits the metabolism of irinotecan, which leads to an increase in exposure to SN-38
- Anti-retroviral agents : Co-administration of delvairdine and saquinavir with paclitaxel has resulted in severe paclitaxel toxicity (CYP3A inhibition?)
- Corticosteroids : decrease the anti-tumour efficacy of aldesleukin
- Herbal supplements: St John's wort decreases the plasma concentration of imatinib and SN-38
- Analgesics: NSAIDs block the elimination of MTX through renal tubular secretion, which results in elevated MTX levels

Drug monographs A–Z

Abiraterone acetate

Zytiga® (prescription-only medicine (POM))
- Tablets: 250mg.

Indications
- Treatment of metastatic castration resistant prostate cancer that has progressed on or after docetaxel chemotherapy.

Contraindications and precautions
- Avoid in patients with moderate hepatic impairment (Child–Pugh Class B).
- Use with caution in patients with severe renal impairment and patients with a history of cardiovascular disease.
- Serum transaminases should be measured at baseline, every 2 weeks for the first 3 months of treatment and then monthly thereafter.
- Blood pressure and serum K^+ should be monitored monthly.

☺ Undesirable effects
Common
- Hypertension
- Hypokalaemia
- Peripheral oedema.

Uncommon
- ↑ alanine aminotransferase (ALT)
- Atrial fibrillation/arrhythmia
- Cardiac failure/angina
- Hypertriglyceridaemia
- Osteoporosis.

Rare
- Adrenal insufficiency.

Drug interactions
Pharmacokinetic
- Abiraterone is a substrate of CYP3A4. Therefore concurrent therapy with strong inhibitors or inducers of CYP3A4 should be avoided, or used with caution.

Pharmacodynamic
- Co-administration with luteinizing hormone-releasing hormone (LHRH) agonists reduces serum testosterone to undetectable levels.
- Co-administration with a corticosteroid suppresses adrenocorticotropic hormone (ACTH) drive and so counteracts the ↑ mineralocorticoid levels that result from abiraterone-induced inhibition of CYP17, resulting in fewer side effects.

⚗ Dose
- 1000mg by mouth (PO) once a day (OD), with concurrent low-dose prednisolone 10mg PO OD.

♪ Dose adjustments
- Interrupt dosing if ALT/aspartate aminotransferase (AST) >5× upper limit of normal (ULN).
- Can resume treatment once LFTs return to baseline, with dose reduction to 500mg OD.
- If significant toxicity on 500mg OD, treatment should be discontinued.

Additional information
- Patients should be fasted for at least 2 hours before taking abiraterone and 1 hour after. Tablets should be swallowed whole with water.

⊕ Pharmacology
Abiraterone acetate is converted *in vivo* into abiraterone, which is an androgen biosynthesis inhibitor. Abiraterone selectively inhibits the enzyme 17α-hydroxylase/C17,20-lyase (CYP17), which is responsible for catalysing the conversion of pregnenolone and progesterone into testosterone precursors dehydroepiandrosterone (DHEA) and androstenedione respectively. Abiraterone therefore acts on the testes, adrenals, and the tumour itself to suppress production of the androgens responsible for driving prostate cancer growth. The half-life of the drug is about 15 hours, with the majority being excreted in faeces.

Alemtuzumab

MabCampath® (POM)
- 30mg vials containing 30mg/ml concentrate for IV infusion.
- May also be used subcutaneously.

Indications
- Chronic lymphocytic leukaemia (CLL) in which fludarabine-containing chemotherapy is not appropriate.
- ¥ First line treatment for CLL harbouring a p53 mutation.
- ¥ First-line treatment for T-prolymphocytic leukaemia.
- ¥ As part of conditioning for allogeneic stem cell transplantation.

NB The licence is about to change as the company that makes MabCampath® is not planning on retaining its haematology licence. The drug will only be available on a named patient basis.

Contraindications and precautions
- Profoundly immunosuppressive—recommended to use prophylaxis with co-trimoxazole (to prevent pneumocystis), an antiherpes agent such as aciclovir, and to monitor cytomegalovirus (CMV) copy numbers with regular PCR testing.
- Avoid in patients with active infections.
- It is recommended that patients should not receive live vaccines for 12 months following treatment.

☹ Undesirable effects
Common
- Hypotension.
- Infusional reactions: fever, rigors, rash.
- Myelosuppression
- Nausea
- Profound immunosuppression resulting in CMV reactivation (which may require pre-emptive therapy) and other opportunistic infections.

Uncommon
- Cardiac arrhythmia.
- Cytokine release syndrome characterized by bronchospasm, angio-oedema, fevers, chills, rigors
- Delayed-onset neutropenia
- Myalgia
- Vomiting.

Rare
- Anaphylaxis.

Drug interactions
Pharmacokinetic
- No significant interactions.

Pharmacodynamic
- No significant interactions.

♪ Dose

Standard dose for CLL is 30mg 3 times a week for 12 weeks. The starting dose is usually lower and escalates during the first week.

♦ Pharmacology

Alemtuzumab is a humanized anti-CD52 antibody. CD52 is widely expressed on cells of the immune system including T cells, B cells, and dendritic cells. Cell lysis is then mediated via complement fixation and antibody-dependent cell cytotoxicity.

Amsacrine

Amsidine® (POM)
- Concentrate for IV infusion, 5mg/ml.

Indications
- Used as part of combination regimens in acute myeloid leukaemia (AML).

Contraindications and precautions
- Careful monitoring and correction of electrolytes needed due to risk of serious arrhythmias with hypokalaemia.
- Fertility:
  - Advise barrier contraception during and for 3 months after therapy.
  - Risk of sterility—advise sperm storage for men.

☺ Undesirable effects
Common
- Fatigue
- Infections
- Mucositis
- Myelosuppression: anaemia, leucopenia, thrombocytopenia
- Nausea/vomiting
- Reduced fertility.

Uncommon
- Abdominal pain
- Diarrhoea
- Hepatotoxicity
- Phlebitis.

Rare
- Cardiac arrhythmias (especially in the context of deranged electrolytes)
- Cardiomyopathy with heart failure.

Drug interactions
Pharmacokinetic
- Amsacrine does not interact widely with other drugs.

Pharmacodynamic
- Myelosuppressive effect potentiated by other myelosuppressive drugs.

⚗ Dose
Regimen specific.

⚖ **Dose adjustments**

Reduction in dose is recommended in both renal and liver impairment. For example, CrCl <60ml/min, reduce dose by 20%; bilirubin >30 micromol/L, reduce dose by 40%.

❧ **Pharmacology**

Intercalates with DNA interfering with replication and transcription. Also specifically inhibits the action of topoisomerase II.

Anastrozole

Arimidex® (POM)
- Tablet: 1mg (28).

Indications
- Treatment of advanced breast cancer in postmenopausal women.

Contraindications and precautions
- Anastrozole is contraindicated for use in:
  - premenopausal women
  - pregnant or lactating women
  - patients with severe renal impairment (CrCl <20ml/min)
  - patients with moderate or severe hepatic disease.
- Avoid concurrent administration of tamoxifen.
- Asthenia (weakness) and drowsiness have been reported with the use of anastrozole. Caution should be observed when driving or operating machinery while such symptoms persist.

Adverse effects
Very common
- Fatigue
- Headache
- Hot flushes
- Joint pain
- Nausea
- Rash
- Weakness.

Common
- Alopecia
- Anorexia
- Carpal tunnel syndrome
- Diarrhoea
- Drowsiness
- Hypercholesterolaemia
- Vaginal bleeding.

Uncommon
- Altered LFTs (gamma glutamyl transferase and bilirubin)
- Hepatitis
- Urticaria.

Rare
- Erythema multiforme.

Drug interactions
Pharmacokinetic
- Unlikely to be involved in pharmacokinetic interactions.

Pharmacodynamic
- Oestrogens—may antagonize the effect of anastrozole
- Tamoxifen—may reduce the beneficial effect of anastrozole.

♪ Dose
- 1mg PO OD.

♪ Dose adjustments
Elderly
- No dosage adjustments are necessary.

Hepatic/renal impairment
- No dose change is recommended in patients with mild hepatic disease, but anastrozole is contraindicated for use in patients with moderate or severe hepatic disease.
- No dose change is recommended in patients with mild or moderate renal impairment, but anastrozole is contraindicated for use in patients with severe renal impairment (CrCl <20ml/min).

♦ Pharmacology
Anastrozole is a potent and selective non-steroidal aromatase inhibitor which does not possess any progestogenic, androgenic, or oestrogenic activity. It is believed to work by significantly lowering serum oestradiol concentrations through inhibition of aromatase (converts adrenal androstenedione to oestrone, which is precursor of oestradiol). Many breast cancers have oestrogen receptors and growth of these tumours can be stimulated by oestrogens.

Asparaginase

Asparaginase medac® (POM)—from *Escherichia coli*

- Powder for reconstitution, 5000 units per vial—can be given intravenously or intramuscularly.

Erwinase® (POM)—from *Erwinia chrysanthemi*

- Powder for reconstitution, 10,000 units per vial—can be given intravenously, intramuscularly, or subcutaneously. Also known as crisantaspase.

Oncaspar® (POM)—pegylated asparaginase (also from *E. coli*)

- 3750 units per 5ml vial—can be given intravenously or intramuscularly.
- Not licensed in the UK.

Indications

- Treatment of acute lymphoblastic leukaemia (ALL) as part of combination regimen.
- Other non-Hodgkin lymphomas that may benefit, e.g. lymphoblastic lymphoma, natural killer (NK)/T-cell lymphoma.

Contraindications and precautions

- Previous allergic reaction to specific product (can use Erwinase® if previously reacted to Asparaginase medac®).
- Should only be administered in areas with facility to treat anaphylaxis.
- Regular monitoring of blood glucose, LFTs, amylase, activated partial thromboplastin time (APTT), prothrombin time (PT), and fibrinogen are recommended.

☺ Undesirable effects

Common

- Abdominal cramps and diarrhoea
- Coagulopathy
- Fever
- Hepatic impairment (commonly causing raised bilirubin and jaundice)
- Hypertriglyceridaemia
- Nausea
- Pain at injection site.

Uncommon

- Development of antibodies which may reduce the effectiveness of the treatment
- Hyperuricaemia
- Neurotoxicity: confusion, somnolence, agitation
- Pancreatitis
- Rash
- Tumour lysis syndrome.

Rare

- Anaphylaxis.

Drug interactions

Pharmacokinetic
- No significant interactions.

Pharmacodynamic
- Hepatotoxic drugs may increase hepatotoxicity of asparaginase.
- Administration of vincristine very close to asparaginase injection is thought to increase risk of reactions.

↵ Dose
- Regimen specific.

↵ Dose adjustments
- Discontinue in the presence of pancreatitis, severe liver dysfunction, life-threatening allergic reaction, or thrombosis.

Additional information

There is concern over asparaginase-induced thrombophilia. During the period of treatment with asparaginase, levels of antithrombin, fibrinogen, and the APTT should be monitored at least twice. If the level of fibrinogen is <0.8g/L or the level of antithrombin is <70% and/or APTT is >2 × ULN at any time then replacement therapy with fresh frozen plasma should be given.

⟡ Pharmacology

Malignant cells of acute leukaemia and some lymphomas are asparagine dependent as they lack the enzymes necessary to make endogenous asparagine. Depletion of circulating asparagines reduces availability of the amino acid for the cancer cells resulting in an anticancer effect. Pegylated asparaginase has a longer half-life than either non-pegylated form and is associated with fewer side effects.

Bacillus Calmette–Guérin (BCG)

OncoTICE® (POM)
- Powder for instillation fluid for intravesical use: 12.5mg per vial.

Indications
- Treatment of primary or concurrent carcinoma *in situ* of the urinary bladder.
- Prevention of recurrence of high-grade and/or relapsing superficial papillary transitional cell carcinoma of the urinary bladder after transurethral resection.

Contraindications and precautions
- In patients with a positive tuberculin test *and* supplementary medical evidence of active tuberculous infection, BCG treatment is contraindicated.
- Concomitant treatment with antituberculosis drugs is contraindicated.
- Contraindicated in patients positive for human immunodeficiency virus (HIV).

☺ Undesirable effects
Common
- Abdominal pain
- Anaemia
- Arthralgia/myalgia
- Dysuria/cystitis/haematuria
- Flu-like symptoms
- Local irritative bladder symptoms
- Nausea/vomiting/diarrhoea
- Pneumonitis
- Urinary tract infection.

Uncommon
- Hepatitis
- Rash
- Thrombocytopenia/leucopenia
- Tuberculous infection.

Rare
- Confusion
- Conjunctivitis
- Cough
- Epididymitis
- Lymphadenopathy
- Paraesthesia
- Peripheral oedema.

Drug interactions
Pharmacokinetic
- No specific pharmacokinetic interactions have been reported.

Pharmacodynamic
- Antibiotics may reduce the efficacy of BCG therapy, so intravesical therapy should be postponed until the end of antibiotic therapy.
- Immunosuppressants or radiotherapy may interfere with the immune response to BCG therapy, so concomitant therapy should be avoided.

Dose
- Induction treatment: weekly intravesical instillation for first 6 weeks.
- Maintenance treatment: weekly intravesical instillation for 3 consecutive weeks at 3, 6, and 12 months after initiation of treatment. Further maintenance treatment depends on tumour classification and clinical response.

Dose adjustments
- When used as adjuvant therapy after transurethral resection of bladder, BCG treatment should start 10–15 days after surgical procedure and only after mucosal lesions post resection have healed.
- If patient has a urinary tract infection, BCG treatment should be interrupted until urine culture is negative and antibiotics are completed.
- If patient has gross haematuria, BCG treatment should be interrupted until the haematuria has been successfully treated or resolved.

Additional information
- For intravesical instillation, insert a urethral catheter into the bladder and drain the bladder completely. Connect a 50ml syringe containing BCG suspension to the catheter and instil suspension into bladder. BCG suspension must remain in the bladder for 2 hours, after which the patient should void the suspension in a sitting position.
- The patient must not have any fluid from 4 hours prior to instillation to 2 hours post instillation (when bladder is emptied).
- Intravesical BCG treatment may sensitize patients to tuberculin, resulting in a positive reaction to purified protein derivative.
- BCG is a live, attenuated form of *Mycobacterium bovis*. It should therefore be prepared, handled, and disposed of as a biohazard material.

Pharmacology
BCG is a vaccine for tuberculosis. Intravesical BCG treatment therefore acts to stimulate the immune system. The exact mechanism of action is not clear, but this treatment appears to induce a non-specific immune reaction, with a local inflammatory response involving macrophages, NK cells, and T cells.

Bevacizumab

Avastin® (POM)

- Bevacizumab 25mg/ml concentrate for solution for infusion.

Indications

- Bevacizumab in combination with fluoropyrimidine-based chemotherapy is indicated for treatment of patients with metastatic carcinoma of the colon or rectum.
- Bevacizumab in combination with paclitaxel is indicated for first-line treatment of patients with metastatic breast cancer.
- Bevacizumab in combination with capecitabine is indicated for first-line treatment of patients with metastatic breast cancer in whom treatment with other chemotherapy options including taxanes or anthracyclines is not considered appropriate. Patients who have received taxane and anthracycline-containing regimens in the adjuvant setting within the last 12 months should be excluded from treatment with bevacizumab in combination with capecitabine.
- Bevacizumab, in addition to platinum-based chemotherapy, is indicated for first-line treatment of patients with unresectable advanced, metastatic, or recurrent NSCLC other than predominantly squamous cell histology.
- Bevacizumab in combination with interferon alfa-2a is indicated for first-line treatment of patients with advanced and/or metastatic renal cell cancer.
- Bevacizumab, in combination with carboplatin and paclitaxel, is indicated for the front-line treatment of advanced (International Federation of Gynecology and Obstetrics (FIGO) stages III B, III C, and IV) epithelial ovarian, fallopian tube, or primary peritoneal cancer.

Contraindications and precautions

Bevacizumab is contraindicated in the following:

- Hypersensitivity to the active substance or to any of the excipients.
- Hypersensitivity to Chinese hamster ovary (CHO) cell products or other recombinant human or humanized antibodies.
- Pregnancy.
- Recent pulmonary haemorrhage or haemoptysis.

Cautions

Caution should be exercised in patients who have the following pre-existent problems:

- Patients with intra-abdominal inflammation: ↑ risk of perforation.
- Tracheo-oesophageal fistula: permanently discontinue bevacizumab. Other fistulae not in GI tract: consider discontinuation.
- Major surgery: do not start bevacizumab within 28 days of major surgery or in the presence of an unhealed surgical wound.
- Hypertension: control hypertension prior to bevacizumab use as it may aggravate the hypertension and increases the risk of proteinuria
- History of arterial thromboembolism or age >65 years: ↑ risk of arterial thromboembolism.

- Congenital bleeding diathesis, acquired coagulopathy, or patients receiving full dose of anticoagulants for the treatment of thromboembolism prior to starting bevacizumab treatment: caution should be exercised as there may be ↑ risk of bleeding.
- Clinically significant cardiovascular disease such as pre-existing coronary artery disease, or congestive heart failure (CHF): use with caution.
- Renal or hepatic failure: there have been no studies in these patient populations so proceed with caution.

☺ Undesirable effects

Common

- Asthenia
- Epistaxis
- Fatigue
- Hypertension.

Uncommon

- Anaphylaxis/anaphylactoid reactions
- Arterial thromboembolism
- Deep vein thrombosis (DVT)/pulmonary embolus (PE)
- Intestinal obstruction/perforation
- Premature ovarian failure
- Proteinuria.

Rare

- Haemorrhage
- Reversible posterior leucoencephalopathy syndrome (RPLS).

In addition to these effects, bevacizumab does appear to increase the risk of chemotherapy-associated toxicity when it is administered in combination with chemotherapy, e.g. diarrhoea, nausea, vomiting, neuropathy, myocardial infarction, CHF, leucopenia, neutropenia.

Drug interactions

Pharmacokinetic

- No clinically relevant pharmacokinetic interaction of co-administered chemotherapy on bevacizumab pharmacokinetics has been observed based on the results of a population pharmacokinetic analysis.
- No drug–drug interaction affecting the metabolism of the cytotoxic agent has been demonstrated when bevacizumab is co-administered with irinotecan (or its metabolite SN38), oxaliplatin, interferon-alfa-2a, gemcitabine, or cisplatin.

Pharmacodynamic

- Bevacizumab increases the risk of chemotherapy-associated toxicity in many instances as outlined in 📖 Undesirable effects, see above.

⚖ Dose

Always as an IV infusion:

- Metastatic colorectal cancer: either 5mg/kg or 10mg/kg of body weight given once every 2 weeks, or 7.5mg/kg or 15mg/kg of body weight given once every 3 weeks.

- Metastatic breast cancer: 10mg/kg of body weight given once every 2 weeks, or 15mg/kg of body weight given once every 3 weeks administered IV..
- NSCLC: 7.5mg/kg or 15mg/kg of body weight given once every 3 weeks as an IV infusion.
- Metastatic renal cell cancer: 10mg/kg of body weight given once every 2 weeks.
- Epithelial ovarian, fallopian tube, and primary peritoneal cancer: 15mg/kg of body weight given once every 3 weeks.

Dose adjustments

- Dose reduction for adverse events is not recommended. If indicated, therapy should either be permanently discontinued or temporarily suspended.

Additional information

Cases of osteonecrosis of the jaw (ONJ) have been reported in cancer patients treated with bevacizumab, the majority of whom had received prior or concomitant treatment with IV bisphosphonates, for which ONJ is an identified risk. Caution should be exercised when bevacizumab and IV bisphosphonates are administered simultaneously or sequentially. Invasive dental procedures are also an identified risk factor.

Pharmacology

Bevacizumab binds to VEGF, the key driver of vasculogenesis and angiogenesis, and thereby inhibits the binding of VEGF to its receptors, Flt-1 (VEGFR-1) and KDR (VEGFR-2), on the surface of endothelial cells. Neutralizing the biological activity of VEGF regresses the vascularization of tumours, normalizes remaining tumour vasculature, and inhibits the formation of new tumour vasculature, thereby inhibiting tumour growth.

Bicalutamide

Casodex® (POM)
- Film-coated tablets: 50mg.

Indications
- Advanced prostate cancer (in combination with LHRH analogues or surgical castration).

Contraindications and precautions
- Use with caution in patients with moderate to severe hepatic impairment.
- No dose adjustment is necessary in renal failure.
- Contraindicated in women and children.
- Avoid co-administration with substrates of CYP3A4.
- Bicalutamide tablets contain lactose, so should not be given to patients with lactose or galactose intolerance.

☹ Undesirable effects
Common
- Abdominal pain
- Alopecia
- Altered liver function
- Anaemia
- Anorexia
- Breast tenderness
- Chest pain
- Constipation
- Depression
- Dizziness
- Dry skin
- Dyspepsia
- Flatulence
- Gynaecomastia
- Haematuria
- Hirsutism
- Hot flushes
- ↓ libido
- Nausea
- Oedema
- Pruritus
- Rash
- Somnolence
- Weight gain.

Uncommon
- Hypersensitivity
- Impotence
- Interstitial lung disease.

Rare
- Cardiac failure
- Liver failure.

Drug interactions
Pharmacokinetic
- Bicalutamide can inhibit the cytochrome p450 enzyme CYP3A4, so should be used with caution in patients on drugs primarily metabolized by this enzyme. Concomitant use of bicalutamide is contraindicated and bicalutamide should be used with caution in patients on ciclosporin and calcium channel blockers.

- *In vitro* studies show that bicalutamide can interact with warfarin binding: PT should be closely monitored in patients who are also on warfarin.
- Drugs that inhibit oxidation in the liver, e.g. cimetidine and ketoconazole, could inhibit metabolism of bicalutamide and so caution should be exercise if using concomitantly.

Pharmacodynamic
- Cardiac failure has been reported during treatment with bicalutamide plus a LHRH analogue.

Dose
- 50mg tablet once a day PO.

Dose adjustments
- No specific dose adjustments are recommended.
- In about 50% of cases, if there is evidence of disease progression whilst on bicalutamide, withdrawal of drug can result in tumour regression.

Additional information
- Tablets should be swallowed whole with liquid.
- Bicalutamide should be started at least 3 days before commencing treatment with an LHRH analogue, or at the same time as surgical castration.
- LFTS should be checked periodically, particularly in the first 6 months of bicalutamide therapy.
- Periodic monitoring of cardiac function is advisable in patients with heart disease.
- Bicalutamide can reduce glucose tolerance so consider monitoring blood glucose in patients receiving bicalutamide in combination with LHRH agonists.

Pharmacology
Bicalutamide is a non-steroidal antiandrogen that binds to androgen receptors without activating gene expression, thus inhibiting androgen stimulus. Bicalutamide is well absorbed following oral administration, is highly protein bound, and extensively metabolized by the liver (via oxidation and glucuronidation). It is thought that androgen receptors exposed to antiandrogens for long periods can mutate, such that the antiandrogens paradoxically stimulate tumour growth. This is thought to be the mechanism by which withdrawal of antiandrogen therapy can reverse tumour progression.

Bleomycin

Blenoxane® (POM), Bleo-Kyowa® (POM)
- Powder for injection.

Indications
- Testicular seminoma and non-seminoma germ cell tumours (NSGCTs)
- Squamous cell carcinomas of head and neck (HNSCC), external genitalia, cervix, and skin
- Hodgkin and non-Hodgkin lymphoma.

Contraindications
- History of hypersensitivity or idiosyncratic reaction to bleomycin
- Acute pulmonary infection or significantly impaired lung function.

Precautions
- ❶ Risk of pulmonary toxicity:
  - Risk factors include GFR <80ml/min, age >40, and cumulative bleomycin dose of >300,000IU.
  - Discontinue treatment and treat with steroids if symptoms/signs (breathlessness, infiltrates on chest radiograph) not clearly related to coexistent pulmonary disease develop.
  - In suspected cases of pulmonary toxicity ideally limit fraction of inspired oxygen (FiO_2) of supplemental O_2 to 21% to avoid exacerbation of lung damage by high O_2 concentrations (clinical decision).
- ❶ Anaphylactoid reactions:
  - ↑ risk in patients with lymphoma (test dose recommended).
- Fertility:
  - Advise barrier contraception during and for 3 months after therapy.
  - Risk of sterility—advise sperm storage for men.

☺ Undesirable effects
Common
- Alopecia
- Anorexia
- Cutaneous hyperpigmentation/pruritus/rash
- Fever and rigors (onset 4–10 hours post treatment)
- Interstitial pneumonitis and pulmonary fibrosis (potentially fatal).

Uncommon
- Myelosuppression (generally mild)
- Nausea and vomiting (minimal emetic risk).

Rare
- Anaphylactoid reactions (↑ risk in patients with lymphoma)
- Raynaud's phenomenon.

Drug interactions
- Renal excretion of bleomycin ↓ by cisplatin nephrotoxicity: consequent ↑ risk of pulmonary toxicity.

- Risk of Raynaud's phenomenon with peripheral necrosis in combination with vinca alkaloids.

Dose

Monotherapy
- 15,000 units 3× /week or 30,000 units weekly or twice weekly IV or intramuscular (IM).
- Continuous infusion at rate of 15,000 units per 24 hours for up to 10 days, or at rate of 30,000 units per 24 hours for up to 5 days.

Combination therapy
- Various: e.g. 30,000 units weekly in combination with cisplatin and etoposide (BEP).

Miscellaneous
- Test dose (2 units over 15min with monitoring for 1–2 hours) prior to administration of full dose treatment recommended for patients with lymphoma (due to ↑ risk of anaphylaxis).
- ▶ Total cumulative dose of bleomycin should not exceed 400,000 units (many investigators recommend limit of 300,000 units)

Dose adjustments

Age
- Maximum total (T) and weekly (W) doses should be reduced with age as follows:
  - ≥80 years: T 100,000 units; W=15,000 units
  - 70–79 years: T 150,000–200,000 units; W=30,000 units
  - 60–69 years: T 200,000–300,000 units; W=30,000–60,000 units
  - ≤60 years: T 400,000 units; W=30–60,000 units.

Renal impairment
- FDA label recommends dose modification according to GFR:
  - GFR >50ml/min: full dose
  - GFR 40–50ml/min: 70% dose
  - GFR 40–50ml/min: 70% dose
  - GFR 30–40ml/min: 60% dose
  - GFR 20–30ml/min: 55% dose
  - GFR 10–20ml/min: 45% dose
  - GFR 5–10ml/min: 40% dose.

Pharmacology

Bleomycin is an antitumour antibiotic that mediates cytotoxicity via single- and double-strand DNA breaks, inhibition of DNA synthesis, and, less importantly, RNA and protein synthesis. Levels following IM administration are 30–50% those following IV. <1% of circulating bleomycin is bound to plasma proteins. 50–70% of the drug is excreted unchanged by the kidneys; the usual half-life of 2–5 hours is prolonged in patients with renal failure.

Bortezomib

Velcade® (POM)
- 3.5mg powder for solution for injection.

Indications
- Multiple myeloma:
  - As monotherapy in disease progressing after treatment.
  - With melphalan and prednisone as first-line treatment in patients unsuitable for bone marrow transplantation.

Contraindications and precautions
- Bortezomib should not be used in patients with acute diffuse infiltrative pulmonary and pericardial disease.
- Patients with pre-existing severe neuropathy should only be treated after careful risk/benefit assessment.
- Tumour lysis syndrome can occur.

☺ Undesirable effects
Very common
- Constipation
- Diarrhoea
- Dyspnoea
- Fatigue
- Fever
- Headache
- Herpes zoster
- Myalgia
- Myelosuppression
- Nausea/vomiting/anorexia
- Peripheral neuropathy
- Rash.

Common
- Abdominal pain
- Altered sense of taste
- Blurred vision
- Dehydration
- Hyperglycaemia
- Hypokalaemia
- Hypotension (especially postural)
- Neurocognitive effects (anxiety, depression, confusion, insomnia)
- Respiratory tract infections
- Vertigo.

Uncommon and rare side effects include:
- Acute diffuse infiltrative lung disease
- Autonomic neuropathy
- Cardiac dysfunction/ dysrhythmia/failure
- Electrolyte imbalance
- Encephalopathy
- Eye pain/irritation/swelling
- Hepatitis
- Hypersensitivity (including immune complex mediated) reactions
- Pancreatitis
- Paralytic ileus
- Rash/pigmentation/erythema
- Stevens–Johnson syndrome.

Drug interactions
Pharmacokinetic
- Potent inhibitors or inducers of cytochrome P450 enzyme CYP3A4 affect the concentration–time curve (AUC) of bortezomib.

Dose

- Monotherapy: $1.3mg/m^2$ IV OD on days 1, 4, 8, and 11 of a 3-week cycle.
- In combination: $1.3mg/m^2$ IV OD on days 1, 4, 8, 11, 22, 25, 29, and 32 of a 6-week cycle (omitting days 4, 11, 25, 32, beyond cycle 4).

Dose adjustments

- The starting dose of bortezomib should be reduced to $0.7mg/m^2$ in patients with hepatic dysfunction and/or peripheral neuropathy.
- A 25% dose reduction is recommended where grade 3 or 4 toxicity is encountered, or if painful grade 1 or any grade 2 neuropathy develops.

Additional information

- Antiviral prophylaxis should be considered in patients being treated with bortezomib.

Pharmacology

Bortezomib is a proteasome inhibitor. It targets the chymotrypsin-like activity of the 26S proteasome, a large protein complex that degrades ubiquitinated proteins. The ubiquitin–proteasome pathway regulates the turnover of proteins. Inhibition of the 26S proteasome prevents proteolysis and affects multiple signalling cascades within the cell, ultimately resulting in cancer cell death.

Buserelin

Suprefact® (POM)
- Solution for injection: 1mg/ml.
- Metered nasal spray: 100mcg.

Indications
- Prostate cancer—advanced hormone-dependent prostate cancer.
- Pituitary desensitization in preparation for ovulation induction regimens using gonadotrophins.

Contraindications and precautions
- Hypersensitivity to the active substance or any of the excipients is a contraindication.
- Buserelin should not be used during pregnancy or lactation.
- Risk of worsening depression and patients with known depression should be carefully monitored.

☺ Undesirable effects
Common
- Acne
- Constipation
- Diarrhoea
- Dry skin
- Erectile dysfunction
- Hot flush
- Hyperhidrosis
- ↓ libido
- Lower abdominal pain
- Musculoskeletal discomfort and pain
- Nausea
- Vomiting.

Uncommon
- ↓ bone density
- Bone pain
- Cardiac disorders such as palpitations
- Depression
- Drug hypersensitivity
- Glucose intolerance
- Gynaecomastia
- Hypertension
- Injection site reaction
- Mood changes
- Weight increase.

Rare
- Breast tenderness
- Leucopenia
- Pituitary neoplasms
- Thrombocytopenia.

Drug interactions
Pharmacokinetic
- None known.

Pharmacodynamic
- May interfere with effectiveness of antidiabetic medication.

₅ Dose
- 500mcg injected subcutaneously every 8 hours for 7 days, then convert to 1 spray into each nostril 6 times daily.

🎵 Dose adjustments

- No dose adjustments necessary.

Additional information

- Initiation of therapy is with subcutaneous injections for 7 days and maintenance therapy with intranasal administration.
- Disease flare is prevented by prophylactic use of antiandrogen.

⟡ Pharmacology

Buserelin is an LHRH analogue and its mechanism of action is by blockade and downregulation of pituitary LHRH receptor synthesis. Downstream gonadotropin release is subsequently inhibited. Initially, buserelin causes an increase in the amount of pituitary hormones, with a resulting increase in testosterone production. However, with longer administration of buserelin, it desensitizes the pituitary gland leading to reduced stimulation of testosterone secretion and serum testosterone levels fall to castration range.

Busulfan

Myleran® (POM)
- Tablets: 2mg.

Busilvex® (POM)
- Concentrate for IV infusion, 6mg/ml.

Indications
- Induction treatment of chronic myeloid leukaemia (CML; although this has largely been supplanted by tyrosine kinase inhibitors).
- As part of the conditioning regimen of a stem cell transplant.
- ¥ Can be used to cytoreduce in other myeloproliferative conditions such as essential thrombocythaemia.

Contraindications and precautions
- In high doses, consider use of regular benzodiazepines due to ↑ risk of convulsions.
- In high doses, consider use of prophylactic heparin due to ↑ risk of veno-occlusive disease of the liver.
- Monitor LFTs.

☺ Undesirable effects
Common
- Alopecia
- Anaemia
- Febrile neutropenia
- Impaired LFTs
- Leucopenia
- Mucositis
- Nausea
- Thrombocytopenia
- Vomiting.

Uncommon
- Agitation
- Alveolar haemorrhage
- Erythema
- Hepatic veno-occlusive disease
- Second cancers (especially myelodysplastic syndrome (MDS)/AML).

Rare
- Cardiac arrhythmias
- Confusion
- Convulsions.

Drug interactions
Pharmacokinetic
- Itraconazole may impair clearance of busulfan—monitor for toxicity.
- Paracetamol may decrease clearance.
- Myelosuppressive effect potentiated by other myelosuppressive drugs.

℥ Dose

Regimen specific. As part of transplant conditioning, typically 3.2mg/kg/day given in 4 divided doses. For CML induction, up to 4mg daily reduced to 2mg daily for maintenance.

℥ Dose adjustments

Caution in liver impairment.

⊕ Pharmacology

This is a cell-cycle non-specific alkylating agent. It has variable bio-availability raising concerns for oral use during conditioning for stem cell transplantation.

Capecitabine

Xeloda® (POM)

- Capecitabine 150mg and 500mg film-coated tablets.

Indications

Capecitabine is indicated for:

- Adjuvant treatment of patients following surgery of stage III (Dukes' stage C) colon cancer as single agent or with oxaliplatin.
- Metastatic colorectal cancer. It is given as a single agent or, more commonly, with oxaliplatin.
- First-line treatment of advanced gastric cancer in combination with a platinum-based regimen.
- (In combination with docetaxel) is indicated for the treatment of patients with locally advanced or metastatic breast cancer after failure of cytotoxic chemotherapy

Contraindications and precautions

Contraindications

- Patients with rare hereditary problems of galactose intolerance
- Known hypersensitivity to capecitabine
- Known DPD deficiency
- Severe renal or hepatic impairment.

Cautions

Caution should be exercised in patients who have the following pre-existent problems:

- Significant cardiac disease, arrhythmias, and angina pectoris as these can increase the risk of cardiotoxicity.
- Pre-existing hypo- or hypercalcaemia as these may be aggravated by capecitabine.
- Concomitant capecitabine and oral coumarin-derivative anticoagulant therapy; monitor INR carefully.
- Hepatic impairment: carefully monitor in patients with mild to moderate liver dysfunction.
- Renal impairment: the incidence of grade 3 or 4 adverse reactions in patients with moderate renal impairment (CrCl 30–50ml/min) is ↑ therefore a 20% a priori dose reduction should be considered to 1000mg/m^2.
- Elderly populations: grade 3/4 reactions are observed with ↑ frequency in elderly populations. Caution should be exercised.

☺ Undesirable effects

Common

- Asthenia, fatigue
- Diarrhoea, nausea, vomiting, abdominal pain, stomatitis, anorexia
- Palmar–plantar erythrodysaesthesia (PPE).

Uncommon

- Chest pain
- ↓ weight and appetite, dehydration, constipation, dyspepsia

- Hyperbilirubinaemia
- Infection
- Neutropenia, anaemia
- Rash, dry skin, desquamation.

Rare
- Cardiovascular: unstable angina, myocardial infarction, cardiac arrhythmia, thromboembolism
- Febrile neutropenia
- Hypertriglyceridaemia
- Neurological: confusion, memory impairment, balance disorder, coma.

Drug interactions

Pharmacokinetic
- Coumarin-derivative anticoagulants: ↑ warfarin effect.
- Phenytoin: ↑ phenytoin plasma concentrations resulting in symptoms of phenytoin intoxication.
- Sorivudine and analogues: a clinically significant drug–drug interaction between sorivudine and 5-FU, resulting from the inhibition of dihydropyrimidine dehydrogenase by sorivudine, has been described. This interaction, which leads to ↑ fluoropyrimidine toxicity, is potentially fatal.

Pharmacodynamic
- Allopurinol: interactions with allopurinol have been observed for 5-FU, with possible ↓ efficacy of 5-FU.
- Radiotherapy: reduce dose of capecitabine.

∴ Dose

Monotherapy
- Colorectal and breast cancer:
  - $1250mg/m^2$ administered orally twice daily for 14 days followed by a 7-day rest period.

Combination therapy
- Colorectal and gastric cancer:
  - In combination treatment, the recommended starting dose should be $800-1000mg/m^2$ administered twice daily for 14 days followed by a 7-day rest period, or $625mg/m^2$ twice daily administered continuously.
- Breast cancer:
  - In combination with docetaxel, the recommended starting dose is $1250mg/m^2$ twice daily for 14 days followed by a 7-day rest period, combined with docetaxel at $75mg/m^2$ as a 1-hour IV infusion every 3 weeks.

∴ Dose adjustments

Single agent
- Grade 2 toxicity—interrupt until grade 0/1 and then: on 1st occurrence, restart at 100%; on 2nd occurrence, restart at 75%; on 3rd occurrence, restart at 50%; on 4th occurrence, discontinue permanently.

- Grade 3 toxicity—interrupt until grade 0/1 and then: on 1st occurrence, restart at 75%; on 2nd occurrence, restart at 50%; on 3rd occurrence, discontinue permanently.
- Grade 4 toxicity—either discontinue permanently or wait until grade 0/1 and then: on 1st occurrence, restart at 50%; on 2nd occurrence, discontinue.

In combination in 3-weekly regimen or continuously

- Dose modifications should be made according to rules listed for capecitabine single agent and according to the appropriate summary of product characteristics for the other agent.

Additional information

Hyperbilirubinaemia can arise during capecitabine treatment and, when an isolated finding with otherwise normal LFTs, is likely to be due to non-clinically-significant haemolysis and needs to be differentiated from tumour progression; there is no reason to decrease the capecitabine dose as it is unlikely to progress.

Chest pain can occur acutely on starting treatment with capecitabine and can be due to coronary artery spasm: capecitabine must be discontinued immediately. For colorectal cancer treatment, some oncologists advocate the use of raltitrexed in its place.

⧉ Pharmacology

Capecitabine is a non-cytotoxic fluoropyrimidine carbamate, an orally administered precursor of 5-FU. Capecitabine is activated via several enzymatic steps; metabolized by hepatic carboxylesterase to 5'-deoxy-5-fluorocytitdine (5'-DFCR), which is then converted to 5'-deoxy-5-fluorouridine (5'-DFUR) by cytidine deaminase, principally located in the liver and tumour tissues. Further catalytic activation of 5'-DFUR then occurs by thymidine phosphorylase (ThyPase) which is found in tumour tissues, but also in normal tissues. There is evidence that the metabolism of 5-FU in the anabolic pathway blocks the methylation reaction of deoxyuridylic acid to thymidylic acid, thereby interfering with the synthesis of DNA. The incorporation of 5-FU also leads to inhibition of RNA and protein synthesis.

5-FU is further catabolized by the enzyme dihydropyrimidine dehydrogenase (DPD) to the much less toxic dihydro-5-fluorouracil (FUH_2), and eventually via 2 other enzymatic steps to α-fluoro-β-alanine (FBAL), which is cleared in the urine. DPD activity is the rate limiting step and its deficiency leads to ↑ toxicity of capecitabine.

Carboplatin

Carboplatin (POM)
- Solution for infusion: 10mg/ml.

Indications
- Ovarian cancer of epithelial origin
- Small cell lung cancer.

Contraindications and precautions
- Peripheral blood counts and renal function should be closely monitored. Myelosuppression may be more severe and prolonged in patients with abnormal renal function.
- Contraindicated in severe renal impairment (CrCl ≤20ml/min).
- Fertility:
  - Advise barrier contraception during and for 3 months after therapy.
  - Risk of sterility—advise sperm storage for men.

☺ Undesirable effects

Common
- Allergic reaction (<2%)
- Constipation
- Diarrhoea
- Fever without evidence of infection
- Injection site reactions
- Myelosuppression (grade 3 or 4 in 10–20%)
- Nausea
- Peripheral neuropathy
- Reduction in hearing acuity
- Renal impairment
- Transaminitis
- Uncommon
- Vomiting.

Rare
- Febrile neutropenia
- Transient visual disturbances.

Drug interactions

Pharmacokinetic
- Concurrent therapy with nephrotoxic or ototoxic drugs, such as aminoglycosides, vancomycin, and diuretics, may exacerbate toxicity due to changes in renal clearance.

Pharmacodynamic
- When used with other myelosuppressive agents the risk of myelosuppression is ↑.

⚗ Dose
- Therapy is repeated at 3–4-weekly intervals.
- Target area under the concentration-time curve (AUC) is generally 5–7.
- The Calvert formula is used to determine dosage:
  Dose (mg) = [target AUC (mg/ml × min)] × [GFR (ml/min) + 25]

⚕ Dose adjustments
• Initial dose should be reduced by 20–25% in patients with previous history of myelosuppression or poor performance status.

⚕ Pharmacology
Carboplatin produces interstrand and intrastrand DNA crosslinks. Its biochemical properties are similar to that of cisplatin but without a significant incidence of the dose-limiting neurotoxicity and nephrotoxicity experienced with cisplatin. However, there is ↑ incidence of dose-limiting myelosuppression. Carboplatin is excreted primarily in the urine within 6 hours.

Carboplatin has a linear pharmacokinetic profile over the doses used clinically and does not interact significantly with drugs that are commonly used in combination chemotherapy. The systemic exposure to carboplatin is described as the area under the AUC and this often correlates with both toxicity and response. In patients with ovarian cancer an AUC of between 5 and 7mg/ml per min is usually associated with the maximal response rate.

Carmustine

BiCNU® (POM)
- 100mg single-dose vials of lyophilized material.

Gliadel® (POM)
- Implant: 7.7mg.

Indications
- Brain tumours (glioblastoma, brainstem glioma, medulloblastoma, astrocytoma, ependymoma, and metastatic tumours).
- Multiple myeloma (in combination with prednisolone).
- Hodgkin disease and non-Hodgkin lymphoma (as second-line therapy, in combination with other approved drugs).
- As an implant (Gliadel® 7.7mg) in newly diagnosed high-grade malignant glioma or recurrent histologically confirmed glioblastoma multiforme, as an adjunct to surgery/radiotherapy.

Contraindications and precautions
- Patients can experience delayed myelosuppression. Therefore blood counts should be monitored weekly for at least 6 weeks after each dose.
- There is a high risk of pulmonary fibrosis, especially when used in the paediatric setting (with delayed-onset pulmonary fibrosis occurring up to 17 years after treatment). This needs to be given careful consideration when planning treatment.
- Patients should undergo baseline pulmonary function tests, along with frequent monitoring during treatment.
- Patients undergoing craniotomy for glioblastoma and insertion of Gliadel® implants should be monitored closely, in particular for cerebral oedema and intracranial hypertension. Treatment with steroids may be warranted.
- Fertility:
  - Advise barrier contraception during and for 3 months after therapy.
  - Risk of sterility—advise sperm storage for men.

☺ Undesirable effects
Common (>10%)
- Delayed myelosuppression (4–6 weeks after drug administration)
- Fatigue
- Infection/fever
- Nausea/vomiting.

Specific to Gliadel® implants
- Abnormal wound healing
- Alopecia
- Cerebral oedema
- Convulsions/hemiplegia/confusion/somnolence
- Headache
- Rash.

Uncommon (1–10%)
- Diarrhoea
- Facial flushing
- Pulmonary fibrosis.

Specific to Gliadel® implants
- Anxiety/personality disorder
- Hyponatraemia
- Insomnia
- Intracranial hypertension
- Visual disturbance.

Rare (<1%)
- Acute leukaemia/bone marrow dysplasia
- Hepatotoxicity
- Renal toxicity.

Drug interactions
Pharmacokinetic
- No specific pharmacokinetic drug interactions are commonly reported.

Pharmacodynamic
- ↑ myelosuppression has been reported when IV carmustine is administered concurrently with cimetidine.

Dose
- As IV monotherapy 150–200mg/m^2 every 6 weeks.
- A maximum of 8 implants can be placed within an intracranial resection cavity, depending on the size and shape of the cavity.

Dose adjustments
- Subsequent IV doses should be adjusted according to degree of myelosuppression with previous dose.
- Development of cerebral oedema with mass effect may necessitate removal of Gliadel® implants.

Additional information
- Gliadel® implants should be handled with care, using surgical gloves, as exposure to carmustine can cause severe burning and hyperpigmentation of the skin.

⊕ Pharmacology
Carmustine is a 1,3-bis(2-chloroethyl)-1-nitrosourea which acts as an alkylating agent, forming intrastrand crosslinks in DNA, which prevents replication and transcription. Following IV administration carmustine is rapidly metabolized, with an average terminal half-life of about 22min. The antineoplastic effects of carmustine are likely due to its metabolites. Because of high lipid solubility and the relative lack of ionization at physiological pH, carmustine crosses the blood–brain barrier quite effectively. About 60% of IV carmustine is excreted in the urine over 96 hours and 6% is expired via respiration. Gliadel® implants are biodegradable in human brain.

Cetuximab

Erbitux® (POM)
- Cetuximab 5mg/ml, solution for infusion. Colourless infusion.

Indications
Cetuximab is indicated for the treatment of patients with KRAS wild-type metastatic colorectal cancer:
- In combination with irinotecan-based chemotherapy.
- In combination with 5-FU/oxaliplatin chemotherapy.
- As a single agent in patients who have failed oxaliplatin- and irinotecan-based therapy or who are intolerant to irinotecan.
- In combination with irinotecan-based chemotherapy to resensitize patients to irinotecan after they have developed resistance.

Cetuximab is indicated for the treatment of patients with HNSCC:
- In combination with radiation therapy for locally advanced disease.
- In combination with platinum-based chemotherapy for recurrent and/ or metastatic disease.

Contraindications and precautions
- Cetuximab is contraindicated in patients with known severe (grade 3 or 4) hypersensitivity reactions to cetuximab in patients with mutated K-ras-expressing colorectal cancer.

Cautions
- Only patients with adequate renal and hepatic function have been investigated to date (serum creatinine ≤1.5×, transaminases ≤5×, and bilirubin ≤1.5× ULN). Therefore in populations outside these parameters, proceed with care.
- Cetuximab has not been studied in patients presenting with 1 or more of the following laboratory parameters: haemoglobin <9g/dl; leucocyte count <3000/mm³; absolute neutrophil count <1500/mm³; platelet count <100,000/mm³.
- There is limited experience in the use of cetuximab in combination with radiation therapy in colorectal cancer.

☺ Undesirable effects
Common
- Conjunctivitis
- Dehydration, in particular secondary to diarrhoea or mucositis; hypocalcaemia; anorexia which may lead to weight decrease
- Diarrhoea, nausea, vomiting
- Headache
- Hypomagnesaemia
- Mild or moderate infusion reactions
- Skin reactions.

Uncommon
- Blepharitis/keratitis
- DVT/PE
- Interstitial lung disease.

Rare
- Severe infusion reaction leading to cardiac arrest
- Stevens–Johnson syndrome/toxic epidermal necrolysis.

Drug interactions

Pharmacokinetic
- A formal interaction study showed that the pharmacokinetic characteristics of cetuximab remain unaltered after co-administration of a single dose of irinotecan ($350mg/m^2$). Similarly, the pharmacokinetics of irinotecan were unchanged when cetuximab was co-administered.
- No other formal interaction studies with cetuximab have been performed in humans.

Pharmacodynamic
- In combination with platinum-based chemotherapy, the frequency of severe leucopenia or severe neutropenia may be ↑, leading to an ↑ rate of infectious complications such as febrile neutropenia, pneumonia, and sepsis compared to platinum-based chemotherapy alone.
- In combination with fluoropyrimidines, the frequency of cardiac ischaemia including myocardial infarction and CHF as well as the frequency of PPE were ↑ compared to that with fluoropyrimidines.
- In combination with capecitabine and oxaliplatin (XELOX) the frequency of severe diarrhoea may be ↑.

Dose

Prior to the 1st infusion, patients must receive premedication with an anti-histamine and a corticosteroid. This premedication is recommended prior to all subsequent infusions. In all indications, cetuximab is administered once a week.
- The initial dose is 400mg cetuximab per m^2 body surface area.
- All subsequent weekly doses are 250mg cetuximab per m^2 each.

Dose adjustments

- Reduce the infusion rate by 50% for National Cancer Institute Common Toxicity Criteria (NCI CTC) grade 1 or 2 and non-serious grade 3 infusion reactions.
- Immediately and permanently discontinue cetuximab for serious infusion reactions requiring medical intervention and/or hospitalization.
- For severe acneiform rash: 1st occurrence, delay for up to 2 weeks and if improved continue at same dose but if no improvement, discontinue; 2nd occurrence, delay for up to 2 weeks and if improved reduce dose to $200mg/m^2$, but if no improvement, discontinue; 3rd occurrence, delay for up to 2 weeks and if improved reduce dose to $150mg/m^2$ and if no improvement, discontinue; 4th occurrence, discontinue.

Additional information

Advise patients to limit sun exposure during and for 2 months after cetuximab treatment.

⟩ Pharmacology

Cetuximab is a chimeric monoclonal immunoglobulin (Ig) G_1 antibody produced in a mammalian cell line by recombinant DNA technology. It binds specifically to EGFR on both normal and tumour cells, and competitively inhibits the binding of epidermal growth factor (EGF) and other ligands, such as transforming growth factor-alpha. *In vitro* assays and *in vivo* animal studies have shown that binding of cetuximab to EGFR blocks phosphorylation and activation of receptor-associated kinases, resulting in inhibition of cell growth, induction of apoptosis, and ↓ matrix metalloproteinase and VEGF production. Signal transduction through EGFR results in activation of wild-type *KRAS* protein. However, in cells with activating *KRAS* somatic mutations, the mutant KRAS protein is continuously active and appears independent of EGFR regulation. *In vitro*, cetuximab can mediate antibody-dependent cellular cytotoxicity (ADCC) against certain human tumour types. *In vitro* assays and *in vivo* animal studies have shown that cetuximab inhibits the growth and survival of tumour cells that express EGFR.

Chlorambucil

Leukeran® (POM)
- Tablets: 2mg.

Indications
- Treatment of CLL in patients not fit for more intensive regimens—alone or in combination with rituximab.
- Treatment of other low-grade non-Hodgkin lymphomas or in Hodgkin lymphoma, 1st or subsequent lines (alone or in combination, e.g. with prednisolone).

Contraindications and precautions
- Patients who have developed resistance to chlorambucil.
- There may be a cross-reaction between alkylating agents producing skin reactions.
- Fertility:
    - Advise barrier contraception during and for 3 months after therapy.
    - Risk of sterility—advise sperm storage for men.

☻ Undesirable effects
Common
- Fatigue
- Infections
- Myelosuppression: anaemia, leucopenia, thrombocytopenia
- Reduced fertility.

Uncommon
- Nausea, vomiting, oral ulcers
- Secondary MDS or AML
- Seizures.

Rare
- Skin rash progressing to erythema multiforme, Stevens–Johnson syndrome or toxic epidermal necrolysis.

Drug interactions
Pharmacokinetic
- Chlorambucil does not interact widely with other drugs.

Pharmacodynamic
- Myelosuppressive effect potentiated by other myelosuppressive drugs.

⚗ Dose
- Regimen specific. As single in CLL, a typical dose would be 10mg daily days 1–14 of a 28-day cycle.

⚗ Dose adjustments
- Consider modifying if gross hepatic impairment.

◈ Pharmacology

Chlorambucil is a bifunctional alkylating agent of the nitrogen mustard type. Alkylation of DNA leads to impairment of DNA synthesis during replication. The result is cell death. Chlorambucil is metabolized by the liver although resulting metabolites are often active. Active metabolites spontaneously degrade in the bloodstream.

Cisplatin

Platinol-AQ®, Platinol® (POM)

- Solution for infusion: 10mg/10ml, 50mg/50ml, 100mg/100ml.

Indications

- Testicular seminoma and NSGCT
- Carcinomas of lung/oesophagus/stomach/ovary/endometrium/cervix/bladder, HNSCC
- Mesothelioma
- Sarcoma
- Non-Hodgkin lymphoma.

Contraindications

- History of allergy to cisplatin
- Significant renal impairment (GFR <40ml/min)
- Clinically significant neuropathy/hearing loss.

Precautions

- Baseline audiogram indicated in younger patients prior to therapy (i.e. testicular tumours).
- Fertility:
  - Advise barrier contraception during and for 3 months after therapy.
  - Risk of sterility—advise sperm storage for men.

☺ Undesirable effects

Common
- Nausea and vomiting (high emetic risk)
- Nephrotoxicity
- Ototoxicity
- Peripheral sensory neuropathy (↑ risk if cumulative dose >200mg/m^2).

Uncommon
- Electrolyte disturbance including: hypomagnesaemia, hypocalcaemia, hyponatraemia, hypokalaemia, and hypophosphataemia
- Myelosuppression (generally mild).

Rare
- Optic neuritis, papilloedema, and cerebral blindness
- Vascular toxicities including myocardial infarction, cerebrovascular accident.

Drug interactions

- Nephrotoxic drugs (aminoglycosides, methotrexate, amphotericin B): ↑risk of toxicity.
- Ototoxic drugs (aminoglycosides, loop diuretics): ↑risk of toxicity.
- Bleomycin/methotrexate: ↑ risk of toxicity due to ↓ renal excretion.

Dose

Monotherapy/combination therapy

- 50–100mg/m^2 IV over 2–8 hours every 3–4 weeks or 15–20mg/m^2 IV daily for 5 days every 3–4 weeks.

Hydration

- Pre- and post-hydration with 1–2L of 0.9% saline required to induce diuresis and minimize nephrotoxicity.
- Supplementation of fluid with 10–20mmol/L KCl and 4–8mmol/L Mg^{2+} recommended to replace renal losses.
- Urine output should be >100ml/hour prior to cisplatin; mannitol 15–25g may be required to promote diuresis.

Dose adjustments

- Renal impairment:
  - GFR >60ml/min: full dose.
  - GFR 50–60ml/min: 75% dose.
  - GFR 40–50ml/min: 50% dose.
  - GFR <40ml/min: contraindicated/consider carboplatin.
- Hepatic impairment:
  - No dose modification required.

Pharmacology

Cisplatin is a heavy metal alkylating agent which mediates cytotoxicity primarily via generation of intrastrand and interstrand DNA crosslinks. Following IV administration ~90% of the platinum compound is bound to plasma proteins within 4 hours. 90% of the drug is excreted renally, with initial rapid excretion of intact cisplatin (15–25% administered dose) within the first 2–4 hours followed by further excretion (20–80% administered dose) of protein-bound drug over the following 24 hours.

Cladribine

Litak® (POM)
- 5ml vial, 2mg/ml for subcutaneous infusion.

Leustat® (POM)
- 10ml vial, 1mg/ml for IV infusion.

Indications
- Hairy cell leukaemia (1st or subsequent lines)—Litak® and Leustat®.
- B-cell CLL patients who have failed to respond to standard regimens containing an alkylating agent—Leustat® only.
- ¥ Other low grade non-Hodgkin lymphomas 1st or subsequent lines.

Contraindications and precautions
- Highly immunosuppressive (myelosuppressive and lymphotoxic) so ensure no active infection prior to treatment.
- Generally ineffective in disease which has become refractory to fludarabine—not recommended in this situation.
- Fertility:
  - Advise barrier contraception during and for 3 months after therapy.
  - Risk of sterility—advise sperm storage for men.

☺ Undesirable effects
Common
- Causes profound lymphopenia with ↑ risk of opportunistic infections, e.g. *Pneumocystis jiroveci* pneumonia
- Fatigue
- Febrile neutropenia
- Fever—reported in > 70% with hairy cell leukaemia treated with this agent, thought mainly to be drug related
- Myelosuppression: anaemia, leucopenia, thrombocytopenia
- Nausea.

Uncommon
- Acute renal failure
- Diarrhoea
- Failure to collect peripheral blood stem cells for subsequent autologous stem cell transplant
- Peripheral neuropathy
- Rash
- Tumour lysis syndrome.

Rare
- Transfusion-associated graft-versus-host disease.

Drug interactions
Pharmacokinetic
- Cladribine does not interact widely with other drugs.

Pharmacodynamic
- Myelosuppressive effect potentiated by other myelosuppressive drugs.
- Not recommended to be used with other agents requiring intracellular phosphorylation (e.g. antivirals) or inhibitors of adenosine uptake (e.g. didanosine, tenofovir).

Dose
Regimen specific. Typically:
- Litak®: 0.14mg/kg daily for 5 days.
- Leustat®: 0.09mg/kg daily for 7 days continuous IV infusion.

Dose adjustments
Contraindicated in moderate to severe renal failure (CrCl <50ml/min) or hepatic failure.

Additional information
Patients should receive irradiated blood products for life after receiving cladribine to avoid the risk of transfusion-associated graft-versus-host disease.

Pharmacology
Cladribine is a purine analogue that mimics the purine adenosine. Through inhibition of adenosine deaminase it inhibits the ability of the cell to process DNA and repair single-stranded DNA breaks. Due to the high ratio of deoxycytidine kinase to deoxynucleotidase in lymphocytes and monocytes, it is highly selective in killing these cell types.

Clofarabine

Evoltra® (POM)
- 20ml vial, 1mg/ml concentrate for IV infusion.

Indications
- Treatment of ALL in paediatric patients who have relapsed or are refractory after receiving at least 2 prior regimens and where there is no other treatment option anticipated to result in a durable response.
- AML following at least 2 prior lines of treatment (¥ may be combined with cytarabine).

Contraindications and precautions
- Close monitoring of full blood count (FBC), renal function, and liver function is required.
- Highly immunosuppressive—avoid if active infection and monitor closely for signs of infection.
- Fertility:
  - Advise barrier contraception during and for 3 months after therapy.
  - Risk of sterility—advise sperm storage for men.

☺ Undesirable effects
Common
- Fatigue
- Febrile neutropenia
- Headache
- Myelosuppression: anaemia, leucopenia, thrombocytopenia
- Nausea/vomiting
- PPE
- Rash
- Stomatitis.

Uncommon
- Acute renal failure
- Anxiety, depression
- Hepatic dysfunction
- Peripheral neuropathy
- Tumour lysis syndrome
- Veno-occlusive disease of the liver.

Rare
- Capillary leak syndrome
- Systemic inflammatory response syndrome (SIRS)
- Transfusion-associated graft-versus-host disease.

Drug interactions
Pharmacokinetic
- Clofarabine does not interact widely with other drugs.

Pharmacodynamic
- Myelosuppressive effect potentiated by other myelosuppressive drugs.
- Cleared by the kidneys so use with agents which can cause renal impairment is generally not recommended.

Dose
Regimen specific. Typically:
- 52mg/m^2 as single agent, daily for 5 days.
- 40mg/m^2 when combined with cytarabine, daily for 5 days.

Dose adjustments
- 50% dose reduction in moderate renal impairment (CrCl 30–60ml/min); contraindicated in severe renal impairment.
- Little information for patients with hepatic impairment.

Additional information
Patients should receive irradiated blood products for life after receiving clofarabine to avoid the risk of transfusion-associated graft-versus-host disease.

Pharmacology
Clofarabine is a purine analogue which inhibits ribonucleotide reductase and therefore reduces the pool of intracellular deoxynucleotide triphosphates. Incorporation into the DNA chain also results in premature chain termination resulting in inhibition of DNA repair and synthesis.

Cyclophosphamide

Cyclophosphamide (POM)
- 50mg tablets.

Indications
- Wide range of tumours as part of multidrug regimens, especially breast cancer and lung cancer.

Contraindications and precautions
- Cyclophosphamide is contraindicated in haemorrhagic cystitis.
- Use with caution on patients with hepatic or renal failure.
- Avoid cyclophosphamide use in patients with severe infections.
- Mesna may be given with cyclophosphamide to reduce urotoxic side effects.
- It is important to maintain hydration during treatment.

☺ Undesirable effects
Common
- Allergic skin reaction
- Alopecia
- Chemical cystitis
- Fatigue
- Haematuria
- Mucositis
- Myelosuppression
- Nausea
- Rash
- Vomiting.

Uncommon
- Hyper- and hypoglycaemia
- Infertility (which may be irreversible)
- Interstitial lung disease
- Venous thromboembolism (VTE).

Rare
- Bladder fibrosis
- Hepatotoxicity
- Pancreatitis
- Stevens–Johnson syndrome
- Toxic epidermal necrolysis.

Drug interactions
Pharmacodynamic
- Oral hypoglycaemic agents may be potentiated by cyclophosphamide.

⚗ Dose
- As part of multidrug regimens cyclophosphamide is usually given at 50–250mg/m^2 PO OD (rounded to the nearest 50mg).

⚿ Dose adjustments

- Treatment should be interrupted for allergic skin reactions.
- Dosing should be interrupted where platelets fall below 100×10^{12}/ml or white cells below 3×10^{12}/ml until recovery.

⟳ Pharmacology

Cyclophosphamide is converted to an active alkylating metabolite. It also possesses marked immunosuppressant properties. The chemotherapeutic and immunosuppressant activity of cyclophosphamide is thought to be mediated by the cytotoxic intermediates produced by activation by mixed function oxidases in hepatic microsomes. Non-enzymatic cleavage, possibly taking place in the tumour cells, results in the formulation of highly cytotoxic forms of the drug. Cyclophosphamide is excreted mainly in the urine, in the form of active metabolites that can cause a chemical haemorrhagic cystitis.

Cyproterone

Cyprostat® (POM)
● Tablet (scored): 50mg (168); 100mg (84).

Generic (POM)
● Tablet: 50mg (56); 100mg (84).

Indications
● Prostate cancer:
  • To suppress 'flare' with initial gonadorelin therapy.
  • Long-term palliative treatment where gonadorelin analogues or orchidectomy contraindicated, not tolerated, or where oral therapy.
  • Preferred treatment of hot flushes in patients receiving gonadorelin therapy or after orchidectomy.

Contraindications and precautions

● Hepatic toxicity has been reported in patients treated with cyproterone acetate >100mg PO daily, usually after several months. LFTs should be performed before and regularly during treatment. If symptoms of hepatotoxicity occur and are believed to be caused by cyproterone, it should normally be withdrawn.

● Cyproterone must not be used in patients with the following condition:
  • Existing thromboembolic condition
  • Malignant tumours (except prostate)
  • Meningioma or a history of meningioma.
● Use with caution in the following:
  • Depression (condition may deteriorate)
  • Hepatic impairment (see earlier in list)
  • History of thromboembolic disease (may recur with cyproterone)
  • Diabetes (cyproterone can affect carbohydrate metabolism; also ↑ risk of thromboembolic events)
  • Sickle cell anaemia.
● Regular blood counts (as well as LFTs) should be performed due to the risk of anaemia.
● Cyproterone may modify reactions and patients should be advised not drive (or operate machinery) if affected.

Adverse effects
Very common
● ↓ libido
● Erectile dysfunction
● Reduced sexual drive.

Common
● Depression
● Dyspnoea
● Fatigue
● Gynaecomastia
● Hepatotoxicity (jaundice/hepatitis)

- Hot flushes
- Restlessness (usually short-term)
- Sweating
- Weight gain (long-term treatment).

Uncommon
- Rash.

Rare
- Galactorrhoea.

Very rare
- Benign and malignant liver tumours.

Unknown
- Anaemia (long-term treatment)
- Dry skin
- Meningioma (long-term treatment)
- Osteoporosis
- Thromboembolic events.

Drug interactions
Pharmacokinetic
- Cyproterone is metabolized by CYP3A4; at high doses it may inhibit CYP2C8, CYP2C9, CYP2C19, CYP2D6, and CYP3A4.
- Co-administration with drugs that are metabolized by, or affect the activity (induction or inhibition) of this pathway may lead to clinically relevant drug interactions and the prescriber should be aware that dosage adjustments may be necessary, particularly of drugs with a narrow therapeutic index.

Pharmacodynamic
- None known.

Dose
- Suppression of 'flare'.
- 300mg PO in 2–3 divided doses after meals for several days before and several weeks after gonadorelin therapy. The dose may be reduced to 200mg PO in 2–3 divided doses if the higher dose is not tolerated.

Long-term palliative treatment
- 200–300mg PO daily in 2–3 divided doses after meals.

Hot flushes
- Initial dose 50mg PO OD, increasing if necessary to 50mg PO 2–3 times daily (BD–TDS).

Dose adjustments
Elderly
- Usual adult doses recommended.

Hepatic/renal impairment
- No specific guidance is available for use in hepatic impairment. The manufacturer advises caution.
- No specific guidance is available for use in renal impairment, although accumulation is unlikely given the hepatic clearance of the drug.

Cytarabine (cytosine arabinoside)

Non-proprietary (POM)

- 20mg/ml; 5ml, 10ml, or 20ml vials.
- Can be used intravenously, subcutaneously, and intrathecally.

DepoCyte® (POM)

- 10mg/ml suspension for injection: 50mg vial.

Indications

- Induction and consolidation of remission in AML (used in combination or as a single agent).
- Induction of remission in ALL.
- Maintenance treatment in older patients with AML.
- Treatment of high-grade non-Hodgkin lymphoma, usually in combination.
- Intrathecally, in prophylaxis or treatment of CNS leukaemia/lymphoma.
- Liposomal formulation (DepoCyte®) is licensed for treatment of lymphomatous meningitis.

Contraindications and precautions

- Hypersensitivity to cytarabine.
- Caution in patients with pre-existing myelosuppression.

☺ Undesirable effects

Common

- Alopecia
- Anaemia
- Cytarabine reaction: fever, myalgia, rash, bone pain, conjunctivitis (in some cases may need treatment with corticosteroids)
- Fatigue
- Infections
- Leucopenia
- Nausea
- Thrombocytopenia
- Vomiting.

Uncommon

- GI haemorrhage
- Oral ulceration
- Pancreatitis
- Pulmonary toxicity.

Rare

- Damage to the CNS, especially cerebellum (may be fatal).

Drug interactions

Pharmacokinetic

- Cytarabine does not interact widely with other drugs.

Pharmacodynamic
• Myelosuppressive effect potentiated by other myelosuppressive drugs.

Dose
Regimen specific.

Dose adjustments
Consider modifying in moderate renal impairment and/or hepatic impairment.

Pharmacology
Cytarabine is a cell cycle-specific cytotoxic, preferentially affecting cells in S phase. It acts as a cytosine analogue, competing with naturally occurring nucleotides to inhibit enzymes involved in DNA synthesis. Cytarabine is metabolized by cytidine deaminase in the liver but a substantial proportion is excreted unchanged by the kidneys.

Dacarbazine

Dacarbazine (POM)
- Powder or solution for injection/infusion: 100mg, 200mg, 500mg, 600mg, 1000mg.

Indications
- Metastatic melanoma.
- As part of combination therapy for soft tissue sarcoma (STS) or for Hodgkin disease.

Contraindications and precautions
- Dacarbazine should not be used in patients with myelosuppression, or those with severe liver or kidney dysfunction.
- Patients should be given prophylactic antiemetics.
- Fertility:
  - Advise barrier contraception during and for 3 months after therapy.
  - Risk of sterility—advise sperm storage for men.

☺ Undesirable effects
Common
- Fatigue
- Myelosuppression (grade 3 or 4 in 5–15%)
- Nausea/vomiting/anorexia.

Uncommon
- Alopecia (usually only thinning)
- Flu-like symptoms
- Photosensitivity.

Rare
- Confusion
- Diarrhoea
- Elevation of liver enzymes
- Headache
- Hepatic necrosis due to veno-occlusive disease of the liver
- Hypersensitivity reactions
- Rash/pigmentation/erythema.

Drug interactions
Pharmacokinetic
- Dacarbazine is metabolized by cytochrome P450 (CYP1A1, CYP1A2, CYP2E1), and affects other drugs metabolized by the same enzymes.

Pharmacodynamic
- When used with other myelosuppressive agents the risk of myelosuppression is ↑.

⚗ Dose
- As monotherapy: 250mg/m^2/day IV OD for 5 consecutive days every 3 weeks, or as a single IV dose of 850–1000mg/m^2 every 3 weeks.

- In combination regimens: 250mg/m^2/day IV OD for 5 consecutive days every 3 weeks with doxorubicin (STS); or 375mg/m^2 IV once every 15 days with doxorubicin, bleomycin, and vinblastine (Hodgkin disease).

₰ Dose adjustments

- Retreatment is guided by the nadir blood counts in the preceding treatment cycle.
- ¥ A 25% dose reduction is recommended where grade 3 or 4 toxicity is encountered.

Additional information

- Dacarbazine is sensitive to light and should be protected from light during administration.
- Doses should be administered as an IV infusion over 15–30min.

⊹ Pharmacology

Dacarbazine is quickly converted by hepatic metabolism to methyl triazenoimidazole carboxamide (MTIC) and then to the active moiety 5-aminoimidazole-4-carboxamide, and acts by methylating DNA. The most important DNA lesion for temozolomide's antitumour activity is considered to be at the O6 position on guanine, although N7 methylguanine may make a contribution. MTIC is excreted renally and has low protein binding.

Dactinomycin

Actinomycin-D, Cosmegen® (POM)

- Powder for injection; vial contains 500mcg dactinomycin with 20mg mannitol.

Indications

- Wilms' tumour
- Rhabdomyosarcoma/Ewing's sarcoma/Kaposi's sarcoma/osteosarcoma
- Testicular seminoma and NSGCT
- Carcinoma of the endometrium/ovary
- Gestational trophoblastic disease (GTD).

Contraindications

- History of hypersensitivity to dactinomycin.
- Concomitant varicella or herpes zoster infection (may result in severe, potentially fatal, generalized disease).

Precautions

- Risk of radiation recall: use with caution in patients treated with radiotherapy.
- ❶ Vesicant: severe tissue damage associated with extravasation.
- Fertility:
  - Advise barrier contraception during and for 3 months after therapy.
  - Risk of sterility—advise sperm storage for men.

☺ Undesirable effects

Common
- Alopecia
- Myelosuppression (nadir 14–21 days)—dose-limiting toxicity
- Nausea and vomiting (high emetic risk).

Uncommon
- Diarrhoea
- Hyperpigmentation
- Mucositis
- Radiation recall.

Rare
- Anaphylactoid reaction
- Elevation of liver enzymes
- Hepatotoxicity including hepatitis and veno-occlusive disease
- Second malignancies.

Drug interactions

- May interfere with bioassays used to monitor antibiotic levels.

⚗ Dose

Monotherapy
- 1000–2000mcg/m^2 every 3 weeks.
- 12mcg/kg/day IV for 5 days (GTD).

In combination
- 1000mcg/m^2 IV day 1 (testicular cancer).
- 500mcg/dose IV days 1 and 2 (GTD).
- 600mcg/m^2/dose days 1, 2, and 3 of weeks 15, 31, 34, 39, and 42 (osteosarcoma).

Dose adjustments

Hepatic impairment
- Consider dose reduction for hyperbilirubinaemia/transaminitis (inadequate data available to guide recommendations).

Renal impairment
- No dose adjustment required.

Pharmacology

Dactinomycin is an antitumour antibiotic that binds to DNA by intercalation, leading to inhibition of DNA replication and RNA synthesis. Following IV administration, dactinomycin undergoes rapid initial excretion followed by a long elimination half-life of 30–40 hours. Dactinomycin is excreted in bile (up to 50%) and by the kidneys (6–31%).

Dasatinib

Sprycel® (POM)

- 20mg, 50mg, 80mg, 100mg or 140mg film-coated tablets.

Indications

- CML resistant to, or intolerant of, imatinib.
- Philadelphia chromosome -positive ALL.

Contraindications and precautions

- Concomitant H2 antagonists, antacids, or proton pump inhibitor (PPI) therapy may reduce exposure to dasatinib.
- Dasatinib interacts with drugs metabolized by cytochrome p450 3A4.

☺ Undesirable effects

Very common

- Bleeding
- Cough
- Diarrhoea
- Dyspnoea
- Fluid retention, including pleural effusion
- Headache
- Infection
- Musculoskeletal pain
- Nausea and vomiting
- Rash.

Common

- Alopecia
- Arthralgia and myalgia
- Cardiac dysfunction, including pericardial effusion, palpitations, and arrhythmia
- Constipation
- Dehydration
- Depression
- Dermatitis
- Febrile neutropenia
- Flushing, shivers, and chills
- GI bleeding
- Mucositis
- Myelosuppression
- Neuropathy
- Pneumonitis
- Pulmonary oedema
- Sepsis
- Somnolence
- Tinnitus
- Visual disturbance.

Uncommon and rare side effects include:

- Acute respiratory distress syndrome
- Confusion
- Hypotension
- Myocardial ischaemia or infarction
- Pancreatitis
- Pericarditis
- Prolonged QT interval
- Rhabdomyolysis
- Tumour lysis syndrome.

Drug interactions

Pharmacokinetic

- Potent inhibitors or inducers of cytochrome P450 enzyme CYP3A4 affect the AUC of dasatinib.
- Caution should be used when dosing dasatinib with medications that affect stomach pH.

⌦ Dose
- CML: start at 100mg PO OD, escalating to 140mg PO OD if no response.
- ALL and advanced phase CML: 140mg PO OD, escalating to 180mg PO OD if no response.

⌦ Dose adjustments
- Dosing should be interrupted and/or reduced for persistent grade 2 toxicities, and resumed at full dose or with a decrease of 20mg or 40mg/day once these have resolved to grade 1 or better.
- No studies have been performed in patients with impaired renal or hepatic function, but renal insufficiency is not expected to affect clearance of dasatinib.

⦿ Pharmacology
Dasatinib inhibits the activity of the BCR-ABL kinase and SRC family kinases along with a number of other selected oncogenic kinases including c-KIT, ephrin receptor kinases, and platelet-derived growth factor (PDGF)-β receptor. Dasatinib binds to both the inactive and active conformations of the BCR-ABL enzyme.

Daunorubicin

Non-proprietary (POM)
- 20mg vial: powder for reconstitution.
- Can only be given intravenously through fast running drip.

Indications
- AML.
- ALL.
- Liposomal formulation licensed for acquired immune deficiency syndrome (AIDS)-related Kaposi's sarcoma.

Contraindications and precautions
- Patients with myocardial insufficiency or history of severe arrhythmia.
- Patient with ongoing myelosuppression or active infection.
- Avoid if previous treatment with maximum cumulative doses of other daunorubicin or other anthracyclines.
- Fertility:
  - Advise barrier contraception during and for 3 months after therapy
  - Risk of sterility—advise sperm storage for men.

☺ Undesirable effects
Common
- Alopecia
- Mucositis
- Myelosuppression
- Nausea
- Rash
- Red colouration of urine for 1–2 days post infusion
- Severe tissue necrosis if extravasation occurs.

Uncommon
- Acute arrhythmia
- Cardiomyopathy with cardiac failure.

Rare
- Anaphylaxis
- Nephritic syndrome.

Drug interactions
Pharmacokinetic
- Daunorubicin does not interact with many other drugs.

Pharmacodynamic
- Myelosuppressive effect potentiated by other myelosuppressive drugs.
- Associated mucositis may interfere with absorption of concurrently used oral medications.

⚕ Dose
- Regimen specific.
- Typical dose when used in AML induction in combination with cytarabine is 50mg/m^2.

☆ Dose adjustments

Doses should be reduced in the setting of raised creatinine or raised bilirubin. Avoid using in severe renal and/or hepatic impairment. Typical modification is to reduce dose by 25% when creatinine >105micromol/L and by 50% when creatinine >265micromol/L.

Additional information

Anthracycline-induced cardiomyopathy is ↑ in the presence of reduced ejection fraction before treatment, hypertension, increasing age, previous mediastinal irradiation, and cumulative dose >550mg/m^2.

⚙ Pharmacology

Intercalates with DNA preventing action of topoisomerase II and therefore inhibiting DNA replication. Although works best in S phase, daunorubicin is not strictly cell cycle specific. Rapid clearance by liver to active metabolites. Biliary and urinary excretion both important.

Diethylstilbestrol

Generic (POM)
• Tablet: 1mg (28); 5mg (28).

Indications
• Palliation of prostate cancer.
• Palliation of breast cancer in postmenopausal women (uncommon).

Contraindications and precautions

> There is a significant increase in risk of DVT with diethylstilbestrol treatment and patients should be reviewed for the need for concurrent antiplatelet/anticoagulant therapy.

• Diethylstilbestrol is contraindicated for use in patients with cardiovascular or cerebrovascular disorder or a history of:
  • hyperlipoproteinaemia
  • moderate to severe hypertension
  • oestrogen-dependent neoplasms
  • porphyria
  • premenopausal carcinoma of the breast
  • severe or active liver disease
  • thromboembolism
  • undiagnosed vaginal bleeding.
• It should be used with caution in patients with:
  • cardiac failure
  • cholelithiasis
  • cholestatic jaundice (or history of)
  • contact lenses
  • depression
  • diabetes (glucose tolerance may be lowered)
  • epilepsy
  • hepatic impairment
  • hypertension
  • migraine
  • renal impairment.
• Thyroid function tests may be difficult to interpret as diethylstilbestrol may increase thyroid hormone binding globulin leading to ↑ circulating total thyroid hormone.

Adverse effects
The frequency is not defined, but reported adverse effects include:
• Cholelithiasis
• Cholestatic jaundice
• Corneal discomfort (in contact lens wearers)
• Glucose tolerance reduced
• Gynaecomastia
• Hypercalcaemia and bone pain may occur in breast cancer
• Hypertension
• Impotence

- Nausea
- Sodium and water retention
- Thromboembolism
- Weight gain.

Drug interactions

Pharmacokinetic
- Despite extensive hepatic metabolism, there are no recognized pharmacokinetic interactions.

Pharmacodynamic
- Antihypertensives—effect may be antagonized by diethylstilbestrol.
- Diuretics—effect may be antagonized by diethylstilbestrol.
- Tamoxifen—potential antagonism.

Dose

Prostate cancer
- Initial dose 1mg PO OD. Dose can be ↑, as determined by a specialist, to 3mg PO OD.
- Higher doses were previously used, but are no longer recommended.

Breast cancer
- Initial dose 10mg PO OD, ↑ as determined by a specialist to 20mg PO OD.

Dose adjustments

Elderly
- The recommended adult dose is appropriate.

Hepatic/renal impairment
- Diethylstilbestrol should not be used in patients with active liver disease.
- There are no specific dose recommendations for patients with renal impairment. The lowest effective dose should be used.

Additional information
- Ideally, blood pressure should be checked before initiating diethylstilbestrol and should be monitored at regular intervals. Should hypertension develop, treatment should be stopped.

Pharmacology
Diethylstilbestrol is a synthetic oestrogen and it binds to an intracellular receptor protein within the cytoplasm when it is transported to the nucleus of the cell. It then has an action on mRNA and associated protein synthesis. Its action in palliative treatment is not completely understood. Diethylstilbestrol is readily absorbed from the GI tract. It is slowly metabolized in the liver to 3 metabolites; CYP2A6 may be involved in this process. Further metabolism to glucuronides occurs. Excretion is mainly via the kidneys and gall bladder (enterohepatic circulation may occur).

Docetaxel

Docetaxel (POM)
- 10mg/L, 20mg/L, or 40mg/ml concentrate for solution for infusion in a variety of vial sizes.

Indications
- Breast cancer:
  - In combination with doxorubicin and cyclophosphamide for the adjuvant treatment of patients with operable disease.
  - In combination with doxorubicin or trastuzumab (tumours overexpressing HER2) for the treatment of patients with locally advanced or metastatic breast cancer who have not previously received cytotoxic therapy.
  - As monotherapy or in combination with capecitabine for the treatment of patients with locally advanced or metastatic breast cancer after failure of cytotoxic therapy.
- For the treatment of locally advanced or metastatic NSCLC in combination with cisplatin (for chemo-naive patients) or as monotherapy after failure of prior chemotherapy.
- In combination with prednisone or prednisolone for the treatment of patients with hormone-refractory metastatic prostate cancer.
- In combination with cisplatin and 5-FU is indicated for the treatment of patients with metastatic gastric adenocarcinoma, including adenocarcinoma of the gastro-oesophageal junction
- In combination with cisplatin and 5-FU is indicated for the treatment of patients with locally advanced HNSCC.

Contraindications and precautions
- Docetaxel should be used at a reduced dose, or omitted altogether, where there is hepatic impairment.
- Patients should be pretreated with corticosteroids.
- Hypersensitivity reactions may occur within a few minutes of starting an infusion of docetaxel, so facilities for the treatment of hypotension and bronchospasm should be available.
- Fertility:
- Advise barrier contraception during and for 3 months after therapy.
- Risk of sterility—advise sperm storage for men.
- Docetaxel should not be given where the neutrophil count is <1500 cells/mm^3.

☺ Undesirable effects
Very common
- Alopecia
- Altered taste sensation
- Anaemia
- Anorexia
- Breathlessness
- Diarrhoea
- Fatigue
- Febrile neutropenia
- Fluid retention
- Hypersensitivity reactions
- Mucositis
- Myalgia
- Nausea
- Neutropenia
- Peripheral neuropathy
- Skin and nail changes
- Vomiting.

Common
- Abdominal pain
- Altered LFTs
- Arrhythmia
- Arthralgia
- Constipation
- GI haemorrhage

- Haemorrhage
- Hyperbilirubinaemia
- Hypertension
- Hypotension
- Infusion site reaction
- Thrombocytopenia.

Uncommon
- Cardiac failure
- Oesophagitis.

Rare
- Bullous cutaneous eruptions
- Interstitial pneumonitis
- Ototoxicity.

Drug interactions

Pharmacokinetic
- Caution should be exercised when administering docetaxel with other cytochrome P450–3A inhibitors, such as erythromycin, fluoxetine, or inducers such as rifampicin, carbamazepine.

Pharmacodynamic
- When used with other myelosuppressive agents the risk of myelosuppression is ↑.

Dose
- Recommended IV dosage: docetaxel 100mg/m^2 (single agent) or 75mg/m^2 every 3 weeks.

Dose adjustments
- Patients with severe hepatic dysfunction should not be treated with docetaxel.
- Granulocyte-colony stimulating factor may be given as prophylaxis against neutropenia, or when this is encountered in previous cycles of treatment.
- Patients experiencing severe neutropenia or severe peripheral neuropathy should receive a dose reduction from 100mg/m^2 to 75mg/m^2 or from 75mg/m^2 to 60mg/m^2 for subsequent doses.

Pharmacology
Docetaxel is an antineoplastic agent that acts by promoting the assembly of tubulin into stable microtubules. Docetaxel also inhibits microtubule disassembly which disrupts essential mitotic and interphase cellular functions.

Doxorubicin

Doxorubicin, Adriamycin®, Rubex® (POM)

- 2mg/ml solution for infusion; 10–150mg freeze-dried powder for injection.

Indications

- Doxorubicin is indicated for a wide variety of solid tumours and haematological malignancies, and is frequently used in combination chemotherapy regimens with other cytotoxic drugs.
- When administered intravesically, doxorubicin has been shown to be beneficial in the treatment of superficial carcinoma of the bladder (T1 only) and as prophylaxis of recurrences after transurethral resection.

Contraindications and precautions

- Contraindicated in patients with myelosuppression and/or severe stomatitis induced by previous treatment with either other antineoplastic agents or radiotherapy.
- Contraindicated in severe hepatic impairment.
- Patients previously treated with maximum cumulative doses of anthracyclines and anthracenediones should not receive doxorubicin. The probability of developing CHF, is estimated at around 1–2% at a cumulative dose of 300mg/m^2 and slowly increases with total cumulative dose to 450–550mg/m^2. Thereafter, the risk of developing CHF increases steeply and it is recommended not to exceed a maximum cumulative dose of 550mg/m^2.
- Caution should be used in treating patients with current or previous history of cardiac impairment
- *For intravesical use,* doxorubicin is contraindicated in patients with urinary tract infections, inflammation of the bladder, haematuria, or catheterization problems.

☺ Undesirable effects

Very common

- Acute arrhythmias
- Alopecia
- Anaemia
- Atrioventricular block.
- CHF
- Delayed left ventricular dysfunction
- Diarrhoea
- Fever
- GI disturbance
- Leucopenia
- Mucositis
- Nausea
- Neutropenia
- Oesophagitis
- Pericarditis
- Photosensitivity
- Red coloration of urine
- Skin reddening
- Stomatitis
- Thrombocytopenia
- Vomiting.

Common

- Anorexia
- Chemical cystitis, sometimes haemorrhagic, following intravesical administration
- Dysuria

- Haemorrhage
- Itching
- Local hypersensitivity reactions in radiation fields
- Septicaemia.

Uncommon
- Acute leukaemia (delayed)
- Dehydration
- GI haemorrhage
- Phlebitis
- Ulceration of the mucous membranes in the alimentary tract.

Rare
- Anaphylaxis
- Conjunctivitis
- Dizziness
- Exanthema
- Hyperpigmentation of skin and nails
- Injection site reactions
- Onycholysis
- Secondary leukaemia when in combination with antineoplastic drugs which damage DNA
- Shivering
- Urticaria.

Very rare
- Acute renal failure
- Amenorrhoea
- Azoospermia
- Hot flushes
- Hyperpigmentation of the oral mucous membrane
- Oligospermia
- PPE
- Thromboembolism.

Not known
- Actinic keratosis
- Arthralgia
- Hepatotoxicity.
- ↑ lachrymation
- Pneumonitis
- Radiation damage that is already healing may reappear following doxorubicin administration.

Extravasation

Perivenous misinjection results in local necrosis and thrombophlebitis. If extravasation occurs, the infusion or injection should be stopped at once. Cooling the area for 24 hours can reduce the discomfort. The patient should be carefully monitored for several weeks. Surgical measures may be necessary. Dexrazoxane infusions or dimethylsulfoxide (DMSO) locally can be considered.

Drug interactions

Pharmacokinetic

- Doxorubicin undergoes metabolism via cytochrome P450 (CYP450) and is a substrate for the P-gp transporter. Concomitant administration of inhibitors or inducers of CYP450 and/or inhibitors of P-gp can lead to changes in plasma concentrations of doxorubicin.
- Paclitaxel administered before doxorubicin may decrease clearance and increase plasma concentrations of doxorubicin. This interaction may be less pronounced when doxorubicin is administered before paclitaxel.
- Doxorubicin may increase serum uric acid; therefore dose adjustment of uric acid-lowering agents may be necessary.

Pharmacodynamic

- Anthracyclines including doxorubicin should not be administered in combination with other cardiotoxic agents (e.g. trastuzumab) unless the patient's cardiac function is closely monitored.
- Vaccination with a live vaccine should be avoided in patients receiving doxorubicin. During treatment with doxorubicin hydrochloride patients should avoid contact with recently polio-vaccinated persons.
- Doxorubicin is a potent radiosensitizer and recall phenomena induced by the drug may be life threatening. Any preceding, concomitant, or subsequent radiation therapy may increase the cardiotoxicity or hepatotoxicity of doxorubicin.

Dose

Monotherapy (IV administration)

- $60–75 mg/m^2$ is recommended every 3 weeks.

Combination regimen (IV administration)

- $30–60 mg/m^2$ every 3–4 weeks, when administered in combination with other antitumour agents with overlapping toxicity.

Intravesical administration

- 30–50mg in 25–50ml of physiological saline per instillation. The optimal concentration is about 1mg/ml. The solution should remain in the bladder for 1–2 hours. The instillation may be repeated with an interval of 1 week to 1 month, dependent on whether the treatment is therapeutic or prophylactic.

Dose adjustments

- In patients, who cannot receive the full dose due to poor performance status, immunosuppression, or old age an alternative dosage is $15–20 mg/m^2$ per week.
- With impaired liver function the dose should be reduced based on serum bilirubin levels: 20–50micromol/L, 50% dose reduction. 50–85micromol/L, 75% dose reduction. >85micromol/L, omit.
- In cases of renal insufficiency with a GFR <10ml/min, 75% of the calculated dose should be administered.
- Dose reductions of 20–50% should be considered for patients experiencing grade 3–4 haematological or non-haematological toxicities.

✣ Pharmacology

- Doxorubicin is an anthracycline antibiotic. The mechanisms of action include a deleterious effect on DNA synthesis via intercalation into DNA (inhibition of RNA and DNA polymerases), inhibition of the enzyme topoisomerase II, and formation of reactive oxygen species (ROS), which can also cause DNA strand breaks.
- Following IV injection, doxorubicin is rapidly cleared from the blood, and widely distributed into tissues. Doxorubicin does not cross the blood–brain barrier. Doxorubicin is rapidly distributed into the ascites, where it reaches higher concentrations than in plasma. Doxorubicin is secreted into breast milk.
- Doxorubicin undergoes rapid metabolism in the liver. The main metabolite is the pharmacologically active doxorubicinol.

Epirubicin

Ellence®, Pharmorubicin®, Farmorubicin® (POM)

- 5ml, 25ml, 50ml, or 100ml of sterile solution of epirubicin hydrochloride 2mg/ml.

Indications

- Breast, ovarian, gastric, lung, and colorectal carcinomas
- Malignant lymphomas
- Leukaemias
- Multiple myeloma.

When administered intravesically:

- Papillary transitional cell carcinoma of the bladder
- Carcinoma *in situ*
- Prophylaxis of recurrences after transurethral resection.

Contraindications and precautions

- Epirubicin is contraindicated in patients with severe hepatic impairment.
- Patients previously treated with maximum cumulative doses of epirubicin and/or other anthracyclines and anthracenediones.
- Patients with current or previous history of cardiac impairment.
- For intravesical use, epirubicin is contraindicated in patients with urinary tract infections, inflammation of the bladder, invasive tumours penetrating the bladder, or catheterization problems.

☺ Undesirable effects

Very common

- Alopecia
- Anaemia
- Febrile neutropenia

- Leucopenia
- Neutropenia
- Red coloration of urine.

Common

- Anorexia
- Chemical cystitis (following intravesical administration) Dehydration
- Diarrhoea
- Hot flushes
- Infection

- Infusion site erythema
- Mucositis
- Nausea
- Oesophagitis
- Stomatitis
- Vomiting.

Uncommon

- Phlebitis
- Thrombocytopenia

- Thrombophlebitis.

Rare

- Acute lymphocytic leukaemia, acute myelogenous leukaemia
- Amenorrhoea
- Anaphylaxis
- Arrhythmia
- Asthenia

- Azoospermia
- Cardiomyopathy
- Changes in transaminase levels
- CHF
- Chills
- Dizziness

- Electrocardiogram (ECG) abnormalities
- Fever

- Hyperuricaemia
- Malaise
- Urticaria.

Not known
- Asymptomatic drops in left ventricular ejection fraction (LVEF)
- Conjunctivitis
- Flushes
- Haemorrhage
- Hypersensitivity to irradiated skin (radiation-recall reaction)

- Itching
- Local skin toxicity
- Photosensitivity
- Pneumonia
- Rash
- Septic shock
- Skin and nail hyperpigmentation
- Thromboembolism.

Epirubicin can be used in combination with other anticancer agents but patients should be monitored for additive toxicity. Additive toxicity may occur especially with regard to bone marrow/haematological and GI effects.

Extravasation
- Extravasation of epirubicin from the vein during IV administration may cause local pain, severe tissue lesions (vesication, severe cellulitis), and necrosis. Venous sclerosis may result from injection into small vessels or repeated injections into the same vein.

Drug interactions
Pharmacokinetic
- Cimetidine given prior to epirubicin increases AUC and should be discontinued during treatment.
- Quinine may accelerate the initial distribution of epirubicin from blood into the tissues.
- Interferon alfa-2b may reduce the total clearance of epirubicin.
- Paclitaxel and docetaxel pretreatment can cause ↑ plasma concentrations of epirubicin and its metabolites.

Pharmacodynamic
- Anthracyclines including epirubicin should not be administered in combination with other cardiotoxic agents unless the patient's cardiac function is closely monitored.
- Vaccination with a live vaccine should be avoided in patients receiving epirubicin.

⚕ Dose
Monotherapy (IV administration)
- Ranging from 60–135mg/m^2 every 3–4 weeks, or 45mg/m^2 day 1, 2, and 3 every 3 weeks, according to the indication.

Combination therapy (IV administration)
- Breast cancer and ovarian cancer: 25–120mg/m^2 day 1, every 3 weeks, according to the indication and regimen.

Intravesical administration
- Bladder cancer:
- Superficial bladder cancer: 8 weekly instillations of 50mg/50ml.
- Carcinoma *in situ*: 50mg/50ml or 80mg/50ml. Prophylaxis: 50mg/50ml weekly for 4 weeks then monthly for 11 months.

Dose adjustments
- In patients with impaired liver function the dose should be reduced based on serum bilirubin levels as follows:
- Serum bilirubin 24–51micromol/L, 50% dose reduction.
- Serum bilirubin >51micromol/L, 75% dose reduction.
- Moderate renal impairment does not appear to require a dose reduction in view of the limited amount of epirubicin excreted by this route. For patients with ↑ serum creatinine levels (>5mg/dl) a dosage reduction is necessary.
- Dose reductions of 20–50% should be considered for patients experiencing grade 3–4 haematological or non-haematological toxicities.
- If local toxicity is observed after intravesical instillation a dose reduction to 30mg/50ml is advised.

Pharmacology
The mechanism of action of epirubicin is related to its ability to bind to DNA. Cell culture studies have shown rapid cell penetration, localization in the nucleus, and inhibition of nucleic acid synthesis and mitosis.

Epirubicin is eliminated mainly through the liver; high plasma clearance values indicate that this slow elimination is due to extensive tissue distribution. Urinary excretion accounts for ~9–10% of the administered dose in 48 hours. Biliary excretion represents the major route of elimination, about 40% of the administered dose being recovered in the bile in 72 hours. The drug does not cross the blood–brain barrier.

Eribulin

Halaven® (POM)

• 0.44mg/ml solution for injection.

Indications

• Locally advanced or metastatic breast cancer progressing after at least 2 chemotherapeutic regimens for advanced disease, including an anthracycline and a taxane unless patients were not suitable for these treatments.

Contraindications and precautions

• Eribulin is contraindicated in patients with hypersensitivity to the active substance or to any of the excipients.
• QT prolongation has been observed with eribulin. ECG monitoring is recommended if therapy is initiated in patients with CHF, bradyarrhythmias, medicinal products known to prolong the QT interval, and electrolyte abnormalities.
• Hypokalaemia or hypomagnesaemia should be corrected prior to initiating eribulin and these electrolytes should be monitored periodically during therapy.
• Eribulin should be avoided in patients with congenital long QT syndrome.

☺ Undesirable effects

Very common

• Alopecia
• Arthralgia
• Asthenia
• Constipation
• ↓ appetite
• Diarrhoea
• Fatigue
• Headache
• Myalgia
• Myelosuppression
• Nausea and vomiting
• Peripheral neuropathy
• Pyrexia.

Common

• Abdominal symptoms including pain/reflux
• Depression
• Dizziness
• Dry mouth
• Dyspnoea and cough
• Electrolyte disturbance
• Epistaxis
• Febrile neutropenia
• Hot flushes
• Infection
• Influenza like symptoms
• Insomnia
• Itching
• Lethargy
• Mouth ulceration
• Muscle weakness
• Musculoskeletal pain
• Oropharyngeal pain
• Other neurotoxicity
• Peripheral oedema
• Raised liver transaminases
• Rash
• Rhinorrhoea
• Stomatitis
• Tachycardia
• Thrombocytopenia
• Vertigo
• Weight loss.

Uncommon

- Angio-oedema
- Dysuria
- Haematuria
- Hyperbilirubinaemia
- Interstitial lung disease
- Neutropenic sepsis

- Oral herpes and herpes zoster
- Pneumonia
- Proteinuria
- Renal failure
- Tinnitus
- VTE.

Rare

- Pancreatitis.

Drug interactions

Pharmacokinetic

- Eribulin may inhibit cytochrome P450 CYP3A4. Concomitant use with substances that are mainly metabolized by CYP3A4 should be made with caution and the patient closely monitored for adverse effects.

♪ Dose

- $1.23mg/m^2$ IV on days 1 and 8 of every 21-day cycle.

♪ Dose adjustments

- The administration of eribulin should be delayed on day 1 or day 8 for if absolute neutrophil count $<1 \times 10^9/L$, platelets $<75 \times 10^9/L$ or there are grade 3 or 4 non-haematological toxicities.
- Following G3–4 toxicity, the dose of eribulin should be reduced to $0.97mg/m^2$. A further dose reduction to $0.62mg/m^2$ may be made.
- The recommended dose of eribulin in patients with mild hepatic impairment is $0.97mg/m^2$ on days 1 and 8 of a 21-day cycle. In patients with moderate hepatic impairment the dose is $0.62mg/m^2$ on the same schedule.
- No specific dose adjustments are recommended for patients with mild to moderate renal impairment. Patients with severely impaired renal function (CrCl <40ml/min) may need a reduction of the dose.

⊙ Pharmacology

Eribulin inhibits the growth phase of microtubules without affecting the shortening phase and sequesters tubulin into non-productive aggregates. Eribulin exerts its effects via a tubulin-based antimitotic mechanism leading to G_2/M cell-cycle block, disruption of mitotic spindles, and, ultimately, apoptotic cell death after prolonged mitotic blockage.

The pharmacokinetics of eribulin are characterized by a rapid distribution phase followed by a prolonged elimination phase, with a mean terminal half-life of ~40 hours. It has a large volume of distribution. Eribulin is weakly bound to plasma proteins. Eribulin is eliminated unchanged primarily by biliary excretion. Renal clearance is not a significant route of eribulin elimination (9%).

Erlotinib

Tarceva® (POM)
- Tablet: 25mg (30); 100mg (30); 150mg (30).

Indications
- NSCLC
- Pancreatic cancer (in combination with gemcitabine).

Contraindications and precautions
- Avoid erlotinib in patients with severe hepatic and renal impairment (CrCl <15ml/min).
- Avoid concurrent use of the following drugs:
  - PPIs and H2 antagonists
  - CYP3A4 inducers/inhibitors.
- There is an ↑ risk of GI perforation associated with erlotinib.
- Use with caution in patients with a history of peptic ulcer disease, or concurrent use of NSAIDs or corticosteroids.
- Patients with Gilbert's syndrome (a genetic glucuronidation disorder) may develop ↑ unconjugated bilirubin plasma concentrations because erlotinib is a potent inhibitor of UGT1A1 (a UDP glucuronosyltransferase isoenzyme).
- Use cautiously in patients with pre-existing liver disease or concomitant hepatotoxic drugs (periodic LFTs recommended).
- Smokers should be encouraged to discontinue smoking since the metabolism of erlotinib is ↑ (CYP1A2 induction) and plasma concentrations will be reduced.
- If patients develop acute onset of new and/or progressive unexplained pulmonary symptoms such as dyspnoea, cough, and fever, treatment should be interrupted pending diagnostic evaluation.
- Should patients develop symptoms of keratitis, an urgent referral to an ophthalmologist should be arranged.

Adverse effects
Very common
- Abdominal pain
- Abnormal LFTs
- Alopecia
- Anorexia
- Conjunctivitis
- Cough
- Depression
- Diarrhoea
- Dry skin
- Dyspepsia
- Dyspnoea
- Fatigue
- Flatulence
- Headache
- Infection
- Nausea
- Peripheral neuropathy
- Rash
- Stomatitis
- Vomiting.

Common
- Epistaxis
- GI bleeding (often associated with NSAID or warfarin co-administration)
- Keratitis
- Raised LFTs.

Moderate or severe diarrhoea should be treated with loperamide and a dose reduction in steps of 50mg should be considered. Erlotinib treatment should be interrupted if severe or persistent diarrhoea, nausea, anorexia, or vomiting associated with dehydration develops. Patients who develop a rash should use an emollient regularly. Consider the use of topical hydrocortisone 1% if the rash persists. Patients can develop a pustular rash, but topical antibiotic or acne formulations are not recommended, unless on the advice of a microbiologist. The rash may worsen on exposure to direct sunlight. Patients should use sunscreen or protective clothing in sunny weather. Patients who develop a rash may have a longer overall survival compared to patients who do not develop a rash. Patients who do not develop a rash after 4–8 weeks of treatment should be reviewed.

Drug interactions
Pharmacokinetic
- Erlotinib is metabolized mainly by CYP3A4, although CYP1A2 is also involved. Erlotinib is a moderate inhibitor of CYP3A4 and CYP2C8; it is also a potent inhibitor of UGT1A1 and a substrate of P-gp, although the clinical significance of is unknown.
- Antacids—take at least 4 hours before or 2 hours after erlotinib.
- Ciprofloxacin—plasma concentration of erlotinib may increase (dose may need reducing if adverse effects develop).
- H2 antagonists—take erlotinib at least 2 hours before or 10 hours after H2 antagonist.
- PPIs—avoid combination as bioavailability of erlotinib can be significantly reduced.
- Concomitant administration of CYP3A4 and CYP2C8 substrates is unlikely to cause significant interactions. However, concomitant administration of other inhibitors will be additive in effect and may cause problems with drugs that have a narrow therapeutic index.
- The clinical significance of co-administration with CYP3A4 inducers or inhibitors is unknown. The prescriber should be aware of the potential for interactions and that dose adjustments may be necessary.
- Avoid grapefruit juice as it may increase the bioavailability of erlotinib through inhibition of intestinal CYP3A4.

Pharmacodynamic
- None known.

Dose
- NSCLC: 150mg PO OD taken at least 1 hour before, or 2 hours after the ingestion of food.
- Pancreatic cancer: 100mg PO OD taken at least 1 hour before, or 2 hours after the ingestion of food.

Dose adjustments
Elderly
- No dose adjustments necessary.

Liver/renal impairment
- No specific guidance is available. Use with caution in patients with mild–moderate hepatic impairment; avoid in patients with severe hepatic impairment.
- No dose adjustments are necessary for patients with mild–moderate renal impairment; avoid in patients with severe renal impairment (CrCl <15ml/min).

❂ Pharmacology

Erlotinib is a human epidermal growth factor receptor type 1/epidermal growth factor receptor (HER1/EGFR) tyrosine kinase inhibitor. It inhibits the intracellular phosphorylation of tyrosine kinase associated with EGFR which causes cell stasis and/or death. Erlotinib is metabolized mainly by CYP3A4, and to a lesser extent CYP1A2, to several to several active metabolites and it is predominantly excreted in the faeces.

Estramustine

Estracyt® (POM)
- Gelatin capsules: 140mg.

Indications
- Prostate cancer, especially in cases unresponsive to, or relapsing after, treatment by conventional oestrogens or by orchidectomy.

Contraindications
- Peptic ulceration
- Severe liver dysfunction
- Myocardial insufficiency
- Hypersensitivity to oestradiol or nitrogen mustard.

Precautions
- Use with caution in bone marrow suppression, thromboembolic disease, cardiovascular disease, diabetes, epilepsy, renal or hepatic impairment, and diseases associated with hypercalcaemia.
- Patients with osteoblastic metastases should be monitored for hypocalcaemia.
- Live vaccines should be avoided.

☺ Undesirable effects
Common
- Diarrhoea (especially in the first 2 weeks of treatment)
- Fluid retention
- Gynaecomastia
- Nausea
- Vomiting.

Uncommon
- Hepatic dysfunction
- Hypertension
- Impotence
- Lethargy
- Rash
- Thromboembolic disease.

Rare
- Angio-oedema
- Bone marrow suppression
- Cardiac failure
- Confusion
- Depression
- Headache
- Ischaemic heart disease
- Muscle weakness.

Drug interactions
- Milk, milk products, or drugs containing calcium may impair the absorption of estramustine.
- ACE inhibitors may increase the risk of angioneurotic oedema.

Dose
- 140mg to 1400mg once daily, usually starting at 4–6 capsules (560–840mg) a day.

Dose adjustments
- Dose adjustment is according to response and GI tolerance.

Pharmacology
Estramustine phosphate sodium is rapidly dephosphorylated in the intestine and prostate to estramustine and estromustine, which accumulate in the prostatic tissue. Estramustine has a dual mode of action. The intact molecule acts as an antimiotic agent; after hydrolysis the metabolites exert an antigonadotrophic effect.

Etoposide

Etoposide (POM)
- 50mg and 100mg capsules.

Eposin (POM)
- Concentrate for solution for infusion: 20mg/ml.

Etopophos® (POM)
- 100mg powder for solution for injection.

Indications
- Small cell lung cancer
- Advanced ovarian cancer
- Resistant non-seminomatous testicular cancer.

Contraindications and precautions
- Contraindicated in patients with severe hepatic dysfunction.
- Fertility:
- Advise barrier contraception during and for 3 months after therapy.
- Risk of sterility—advise sperm storage for men.

☹ Undesirable effects
Common
- Alopecia
- Anorexia
- Diarrhoea
- Fatigue
- Hepatic dysfunction
- Myelosuppression (grade 3 or 4 in 10–20%)
- Nausea
- Stomatitis
- Vomiting.

Uncommon
- Arrhythmias
- Mucositis
- Peripheral neuropathy.

Rare
- Constipation
- Reversible visual loss

Drug interactions
Pharmacokinetic
- Phenylbutazone, sodium salicylate, and salicylic acid can affect protein binding of etoposide.

Pharmacodynamic
- When used with other myelosuppressive agents the risk of myelosuppression is ↑.

♣ Dose
- The usual IV dose ranges from 100–120mg/m^2 per day via continuous infusion over 30min for 3–5 days, usually every 21 days.
- Oral administration: dependent on indication. Recommended dose 120–240mg/m^2 daily for 5 days, every 21 days.

♣ Dose adjustments
- Patients with a CrCl of between 15ml to 50ml/minute: 75% of the initial recommended etoposide dose should be administered.

Additional information
- Capsules should be taken whilst fasting, and should be swallowed whole.

♦ Pharmacology
Etoposide is a semi-synthetic derivative of podophyllotoxin, which arrests the cell cycle in the G2 phase. Etoposide forms a ternary complex with DNA and the topoisomerase II enzyme, preventing re-ligation of DNA strands and inducing DNA strand breaks and promoting apoptosis.

Etoposide is ~94% protein-bound in human serum, and urinary excretion accounts for 45% of the administered dose, with 29% being excreted unchanged in 72 hours. It is metabolized by CYP3A4.

Everolimus

Everolimus
- Tablets 5mg, 10mg.

Indications
- Advanced renal cancer progressed on or after treatment with VEGF-targeted therapy.
- Unresectable or metastatic, well- or moderately-differentiated neuroendocrine tumours of pancreatic origin in adults with progressive disease.

Contraindications and precautions
- Co-administration with potent CYP3A4 inducers or inhibitors and/or the multidrug efflux pump P-gp should be avoided.
- Hypersensitivity to the active substance or any of the excipients is a contraindication.

☺ Undesirable effects
Common
- Anaemia
- Diarrhoea
- Dry skin
- Fatigue/asthenia
- Hypercholesterolaemia/hypertriglyceridaemia
- Hyperglycaemia
- Nausea/vomiting
- Stomatitis.

Uncommon
- Arthralgia
- CHF
- Dyspnoea
- Neutropenia
- Pneumonitis.

Rare
- Acute respiratory distress syndrome
- Angio-oedema
- Impaired wound healing.

Drug interactions
Pharmacokinetic
- Everolimus is metabolized by cytochrome P450 (CYP3A4), and is also a substrate and moderate inhibitor of P-gp. Absorption and subsequent elimination of everolimus may be influenced by substances that affect CYP3A4 and/or P-gp.

Pharmacodynamic
- Not extensively studied in combination, *in vitro* and *in vivo* models have not suggested significant concerns.

♪ Dose

- The recommended dose is 10mg OD. Treatment continues for as long as the drug is tolerated with clinical benefit or until the appearance of unacceptable toxicity.

♪ Dose adjustments

- A dose reduction to 5mg is recommended with severe or intolerable side effects.

Additional information

- There is no data with the use of everolimus in pregnancy and it is therefore not recommended.
- Male fertility may be compromised based on preclinical data.

✷ Pharmacology

Everolimus is a signal transduction inhibitor targeting mTOR, or more specifically, mTORC1 (mTOR complex 1). mTOR a key serine-threonine kinase has a central role in the regulation of cell growth, proliferation, and survival.

Exemestane

Aromasin® (POM)
- Tablet: 25mg (30; 90).

Generic (POM)
- Tablet: 25mg (30).

Indications
- Adjuvant treatment of oestrogen receptor-positive early breast cancer in postmenopausal women following 2–3 years of tamoxifen therapy.
- Advanced breast cancer in postmenopausal women in whom antioestrogen therapy has failed.

Contraindications and precautions
- Not to be used in premenopausal women.
- Use with caution in patients with hepatic or renal impairment.
- May cause reduction in bone mineral density and an ↑ fracture rate. Women with osteoporosis or at risk of osteoporosis should have their bone mineral density formally assessed and treatment should be initiated in at-risk patients.
- Exemestane may modify reactions and patients should be advised to not drive (or operate machinery) if affected.

Adverse effects
Very common
- Fatigue
- Headache
- Hot flushes
- ↑ sweating
- Insomnia
- Musculoskeletal pain
- Nausea.

Common
- Anorexia
- Carpal tunnel syndrome
- Depression
- Dizziness
- Dyspepsia
- Fracture
- Osteoporosis
- Peripheral oedema.

Uncommon
- Drowsiness
- Weakness.

Drug interactions

Pharmacokinetic
- Is metabolized by CYP3A4. Co-administration with drugs that are metabolized by, or affect the activity of this pathway may lead to clinically relevant drug interactions and the prescriber should be aware that dosage adjustments may be necessary, particularly of drugs with a narrow therapeutic index.
- The effect of grapefruit juice on the absorption of exemestane is unknown.

Pharmacodynamic
- Oestrogens—may antagonize the effect of exemestane.

Dose
- 25mg PO OD, after food.

Dose adjustments

Elderly
- Dose adjustments are unnecessary.

Hepatic/renal impairment
- No dose adjustments are required for patients with liver or renal impairment.

Additional information
- In patients with early breast cancer, treatment should continue until completion of 5 years of combined sequential adjuvant hormonal therapy (tamoxifen followed by exemestane), or earlier if tumour relapse occurs.
- In patients with advanced breast cancer, treatment should continue until tumour progression is evident.

Pharmacology

Exemestane is an irreversible, steroidal aromatase inhibitor which does not possess any progestogenic, androgenic, or oestrogenic activity. It reduces oestrogen levels by blocking the action of aromatase in the adrenal glands.

Fludarabine

Fludara® (POM)

- 50mg powder for solution for injection.
- Tablets: 10mg.

Indications

- Treatment of CLL in patients with sufficient bone marrow reserve (usually in combination with cyclophosphamide).
- Treatment of other low-grade non-Hodgkin lymphomas, first or subsequent lines (often in combination with cyclophosphamide and rituximab).
- Treatment of AML or ALL (often in combination with cytarabine).
- As part of condition for allogeneic stem cell/bone marrow transplant (part of non-myeloablative conditioning regimen, often in combination with an alkylating agent).

Contraindications and precautions

- Avoid in auto-immune haemolytic anaemia as may make it worse.
- Reduce dose by 50% if CrCl 30–70ml/min; avoid if <30ml/min.
- Avoid if poor marrow reserve.
- Avoid if history of frequent or particularly severe infections.
- Fertility:
  - Advise barrier contraception during and for 3 months after therapy.
  - Risk of sterility—advise sperm storage for men.

☺ Undesirable effects

Common

- Causes profound lymphopenia with ↑ risk of opportunistic infections, e.g. *Pneumocystis jiroveci* pneumonia
- Fatigue
- Febrile neutropenia
- Myelosuppression: anaemia, leucopenia, thrombocytopenia
- Nausea.

Uncommon

- Diarrhoea
- Failure to collect peripheral blood stem cells for subsequent autologous stem cell transplant
- Hyperuricaemia
- Peripheral neuropathy
- Rash
- Tumour lysis syndrome.

Rare

- Pulmonary hypersensitivity
- Transfusion-associated graft-versus-host disease.

Drug interactions

Pharmacokinetic
- Fludarabine does not interact widely with other drugs.

Pharmacodynamic
- Myelosuppressive effect potentiated by other myelosuppressive drugs.

Dose
Regimen specific. Typically 25mg/m² orally daily for 5 days when used in combination with cyclophosphamide and rituximab in CLL.

Dose adjustments
- Reduce dose by 50% if CrCl 30–70ml/min and omit if <30ml/min

Additional information
- Patients should receive irradiated blood products for life after receiving fludarabine to avoid the risk of transfusion-associated graft-versus-host disease.

Pharmacology
Fludarabine is a purine analogue and inhibits DNA synthesis by interfering with DNA polymerase and ribonucleotide reductase. It acts on both resting and dividing cells. It is available as oral and IV formulations. It is excreted renally.

Fluorouracil

(5-fluoro-2,4(1H,3H)-pyrimidinedione; 5-FU.)

Adrucil® (POM), Carac® (POM), Efudix® (POM), Efudex® (POM), Fluoroplex® (POM)

- IV injection: 50mg/ml.
- 2.5g or 5g pharmacy bulk package.

Generic (POM)

- IV injection: 50mg/ml.
- 2.5g or 5g pharmacy bulk package.

Indications

- Principally for GI, breast, and head and neck cancers.

Contraindications and precautions

- General contraindications:
  - Poor nutritional state.
  - Depressed bone marrow function.
  - Potentially serious infections.
  - History of major surgery within the previous month.
  - Known hypersensitivity to 5-FU.
- General precautions:
  - Use with caution in patients with history of high-dose pelvic irradiation, previous use of alkylating agents, widespread bone marrow metastases, impaired hepatic or renal function.
  - Deficiency of dipyrimidine dehydrogenase activity may cause prolonged 5-FU clearance and toxicity.
  - May cause fetal harm.
  - Advise women to avoid becoming pregnant.
  - Potential hazard to the fetus therefore use during pregnancy only if the potential benefit justifies the risk to the fetus.
  - When combined with calcium leucovorin adjust dose accordingly.

☺ Undesirable effects

Side effects vary according to dose and to regimen with neutropenia and stomatitis being commoner when frequent bolus injection is used and PPE occurring more frequently with prolonged infusion.

Common

- Alopecia
- Anorexia, nausea, vomiting, diarrhoea, taste changes
- Dermatitis (principally pruritic maculopapular rash)
- Fatigue
- Leucopenia, thrombocytopenia, anaemia
- Stomatitis, oesophagopharyngitis, mucositis causing abdominal pain.

Uncommon

- Acute chest pain due to coronary artery spasm.
- PPE (redness or desquamation of the skin of the palms or soles).
- Sensitivity to UV rays

- Thrombophlebitis (vein tracking).

Rare
- Cerebellar syndrome
- Memory difficulties.

Interactions
Pharmacokinetic
- Cimetidine: metabolism of 5-FU inhibited by cimetidine.
- Coumarins: 5-FU enhances anticoagulant effect of coumarins.
- Filgrastim: neutropenia possibly exacerbated when 5-FU given with filgrastim.
- Metronidazole (oral/IV): metabolism of 5-FU inhibited by metronidazole (↑ toxicity).
- Phenytoin (oral/IV): 5-FU possibly inhibits metabolism of phenytoin (↑ risk of toxicity).

Pharmacodynamic
- Temoporfin: ↑ skin photosensitivity when *topical* 5-FU used with temoporfin

Dose
- Dosing is according to body surface area. Dose per metre squared depends on whether bolus or infusion 5-FU, and for infusion, what is the duration of infusion and what other drugs are being co-administered.

Dose adjustments
Elderly
- Dose adjustments are not mandatory in the elderly but a 20% dose reduction may be recommended if infirm

Hepatic/renal impairment
- No detailed data but it is likely that 5-FU is safe in mild to moderate renal impairment but a dose reduction should be made a priori with moderate liver impairment and 5-FU avoided in severe hepatic impairment.

Additional information
If coronary artery spasm and acute chest pain do occur with 5-FU, raltitrexed can be used as an alternative agent.

Pharmacology
Fluorouracil is a pyrimidine analogue, working through irreversible inhibition of TS. It belongs to the antimetabolites family of drugs. As a pyrimidine analogue, it is transformed inside the cell into different cytotoxic metabolites which are then incorporated into DNA and RNA, finally inducing cell cycle arrest and apoptosis by inhibiting the cell's ability to synthesize DNA. It is an S-phase specific drug and only active during certain cell cycles. Up to 80% of administered 5-FU is broken down by DPD in the liver. DPD deficiency acutely exacerbates fluorouracil toxicity and increases the risk of toxic death.

Flutamide

Drogenil® (POM)
- Tablets: 250mg.

Indications
- Initial treatment of prostate cancer in combination with an LHRH agonist
- Advanced prostate cancer, either as monotherapy or in combination with LHRH agonists or surgical castration.

Contraindications and precautions
- Hepatotoxicity has been reported with flutamide. Flutamide therapy should not be started if serum transaminases exceed 2–3× ULN. LFTs should be checked regularly whilst on treatment.
- Flutamide should be used with caution in patients with cardiac disease, as it can cause fluid retention.
- Bicalutamide is now generally used instead of flutamide due to having a better side effect profile.

☺ Undesirable effects
Common
- Fatigue
- Gynaecomastia/galactorrhoea
- ↑ appetite
- Insomnia
- Nausea/vomiting.

Uncommon
- Diarrhoea
- Transaminitis.

Rare
- Anxiety/depression
- Bruising
- ↓ libido
- Haemolytic or macrocytic anaemia
- Herpes zoster infection
- Hyperglycaemia
- Lupus-like syndrome
- Peripheral oedema.

Drug interactions
Pharmacokinetic
- When administered concurrently with oral anticoagulants flutamide can increase PT.
- When administered concurrently with theophylline, flutamide can increase theophylline plasma concentration.

Pharmacodynamic
- Concurrent administration with hepatotoxic drugs should be avoided.

Gefitinib

Iressa® (POM)

- Tablets 250mg.

Indications

- Locally advanced or metastatic NSCLC with activating mutations of EGFR tyrosine kinase.

Contraindications and precautions

- Caution is advised when administering gefitinib with strong inducers inhibitors of CYP3A4.

☺ Undesirable effects

Common

- Anorexia
- Diarrhoea
- Mouth ulcers
- Nausea/vomiting
- Rash, acne, dry skin
- Weight loss.

Uncommon

- Alopecia
- Conjunctivitis
- Cystitis
- Haemorrhage such as epistaxis or haematuria
- Interstitial lung disease
- Nail disorders.

Rare

- Aberrant eyelash and hair growth
- Corneal erosion
- GI perforation
- Haemorrhagic cystitis
- Hepatitis
- Pancreatitis.

Drug interactions

Pharmacokinetic

- Gefitinib is metabolized by CYP3A4 and can be affected by co-administration of other drugs that are inhibitors or inducers of CYP3A4.
- In patients with a CYP2D6 PM genotype, treatment with a potent CYP3A4 inhibitor might lead to ↑ plasma levels of gefitinib.
- INR elevations and/or bleeding events have been demonstrated wi co-administration of warfarin.

Pharmacodynamic

- Gefitinib is not licensed in combination with other chemotherapeu drugs.

♣ Dose
- As monotherapy, 250mg PO TDS.

♣ Dose adjustments
- The dose may need adjusting in patients with renal insufficiency.

Additional information
- When used as an initial treatment with an LHRH agonist, flutamide should be started at least 24 hours before the LHRH agonist to reduce tumour flare reaction.
- As an adjunct to radiotherapy treatment, flutamide should begin 8 weeks prior to radiotherapy and continue through the course of radiotherapy.

♦ Pharmacology
Flutamide is a non-steroidal oral antiandrogen which acts to either block the uptake of androgens or inhibit cytoplasmic and nuclear binding of androgen in target tissue. When given in combination with surgical or medical castration, flutamide suppresses both testicular and adrenal androgen activity. Flutamide is metabolized to its active form 2-hydroxy-flutamide by the CYP1A2 liver enzyme. Flutamide has a half-life of about 2 hours and is excreted mainly by the kidneys.

Folinic acid (usually administered as calcium folinate)

Leucovorin, Wellcovorin® POM

- Calcium folinate 3mg/ml solution for injection.

Indications

- Following methotrexate as part of a total chemotherapeutic plan, where it may 'rescue' bone marrow and GI mucosa cells from methotrexate.
- As treatment of acute methotrexate overdose. Folinic acid should be re-dosed until the methotrexate level is $<5 \times 10^{-8}$ M.
- In combination with the chemotherapy agent 5-FU in treating colon cancer. In this case, folinic acid enhances the effect of 5-FU by inhibiting thymidylate synthase (TS).
- To prevent toxic effects of high doses of antimicrobial dihydrofolate reductase (DHFR) inhibitors such as trimethoprim and pyrimethamine.
- In the treatment of toxoplasmosis retinitis, in combination with the folic acid antagonists pyrimethamine and sulfadiazine.

Contraindications and precautions

Contraindications
- Known hypersensitivity to calcium folinate, or to any of the excipients.
- Pernicious anaemia or other anaemias due to vitamin B12 deficiency.

Cautions
- Excessive folinic acid doses must be avoided since this might impair the antitumour activity of methotrexate, especially in CNS tumours.

☺ Undesirable effects

Uncommon
- Fever.

Rare
- Anaphylactoid reaction
- Insomnia, agitation, depression
- Nausea, vomiting, abdominal pain.

Drug interactions

Pharmacokinetic
- When given in conjunction with folic acid antagonists the efficacy of the folic acid antagonist may be reduced or completely neutralized.
- When given with antiepileptic substances, may reduce effectiveness and increase the frequency of seizures; a decrease of plasma levels of enzymatic inductor anticonvulsant drugs may be observed because the hepatic metabolism is ↑ as folates are cofactors.

Dose

Rescue in methotrexate therapy

The methotrexate protocol will dictate the dosage regimen of folinic acid rescue. Refer to the applied intermediate- or high-dose methotrexate protocol for posology and method of administration of calcium folinate. However:

- The first dose of folinic acid is 15mg (6–$12mg/m^2$) to be given 12–24 hours after the beginning of methotrexate infusion. The same dose is given every 6 hours throughout a period of 72 hours. After several parenteral doses treatment can be switched over to the oral form.
- 48 hours after the start of the methotrexate infusion, the residual methotrexate level should be measured and folinic acid dosages should be adapted according to local protocols.

Trimetrexate toxicity

- Prevention: folinic acid should be administered every day during treatment with trimetrexate and for 72 hours after the last dose. It can be administered either by the IV route at a dose of $20mg/m^2$ over 5–$10min$ every 6 hours for a total daily dose of $80mg/m^2$, or by oral route with 4 doses of $20mg/m^2$ administered at equal time intervals.
- Overdosage: after stopping trimetrexate, calcium folinate $40mg/m^2$ IV every 6 hours for 3 days.

Trimethoprim toxicity

- After stopping trimethoprim, 3–$10mg/day$ folinic acid until recovery of a normal blood count.

Pyrimethamine toxicity

- In case of high-dose pyrimethamine, folinic acid 5–$50mg/day$ should be administered, based on the results of the peripheral blood counts.

Enhancing efficacy of 5-FU

- 20mg when administered with bolus 5-FU regimens.
- 350mg when administered with infusional regimen, although the evidence for the use of such a high dose is lacking.

Dose adjustments

- None are stipulated.

Additional information

- IV folinic acid can be administered for the prevention and treatment of folate deficiency when it cannot be prevented or corrected by the administration of folic acid by the oral route.

Pharmacology

Folinic acid is a 5-formyl derivative of tetrahydrofolic acid and is readily converted to other reduced folic acid derivatives. It has activity that is equivalent to that of folic acid but its function is unaffected by drugs such as methotrexate. Folinic acid, therefore, allows for some purine/pyrimidine synthesis to occur in the presence of DHFR inhibition, so that some normal DNA replication and RNA transcription processes can proceed.

- In combination studies with vinorelbine it has been shown to exacerbate the neutropenic effect of vinorelbine.

Dose

- The dose of gefitinib is 250mg PO OD.

Dose adjustments

- For patients with severe diarrhoea or skin adverse reactions therapy interruption (up to 14 days) followed by reinstatement of the 250mg dose may be successful. For patients unable to tolerate treatment after a therapy interruption, gefitinib should be discontinued.

Additional information

- Gefitinib may be taken with or without food. The tablet can be swallowed whole with some water or if dosing of whole tablets is not possible, tablets may be dissolved in water.

Pharmacology

Gefitinib is a selective inhibitor of EGFR tyrosine kinase domain. The target protein (EGFR) is a family of receptors which includes HER1 (Erb-B1), HER2 (Erb-B2), and HER3 (Erb-B3). The metabolism of gefitinib is via the cytochrome P450 isoenzyme CYP3A4 (predominantly) and via CYP2D6.

Gemcitabine

2′,2′ -difluourodeoxycytidine (dFdC), Gemzar® (POM)

- Powder for solution for infusion: 200mg, 1000mg.

Indications

- Carcinoma of the pancreas (monotherapy and combination)
- NSCLC (monotherapy and in combination with cisplatin)
- Carcinoma of the bladder in combination with cisplatin
- Relapsed ovarian carcinoma in combination with carboplatin
- Metastatic breast carcinoma
- Refractory testicular seminoma and NSGCT.

Contraindications

- History of hypersensitivity to gemcitabine
- Breastfeeding.

Precautions

- Potent radiosensitizer: use with caution within 7 days of radiotherapy.
- Use with caution in patients with hepatic or renal insufficiency.
- Fertility:
  - Advise barrier contraception during and for 3 months after therapy.
  - Risk of sterility—advise sperm storage for men.

☺ Undesirable effects

Common
- Diarrhoea
- ↑ hepatic transaminases/alkaline phosphatase
- Mucositis
- Myelosuppression
- Proteinuria/haematuria
- Rash/pruritus
- Transient dyspnoea/cough.

Uncommon
- Bronchospasm
- Interstitial pneumonitis
- Nausea/vomiting (low emetic risk)
- Renal failure.

Rare
- Anaphylaxis
- Haemolytic uraemic syndrome
- Radiation recall
- Thrombocytosis
- Vasculitis.

Drug interactions

- Pharmacokinetics unchanged by administration in combination with paclitaxel or carboplatin.

♣ Dose

Monotherapy

- 1000mg/m^2 weekly for 7 weeks followed by a week of rest, then weekly for 3 weeks out of 4 (pancreatic cancer).
- Weekly for 3 weeks out of 4 (NSCLC).

In combination

- 1000mg/m^2 on day 1, 8, and 15 of a 28-day cycle in combination with cisplatin 70mg/m^2 on day 1 (bladder).
- 1250mg/m^2 on day 1 and 8 of a 21-day treatment cycle in combination with cisplatin (75–100mg/m^2) or carboplatin (AUC 4–5) on day 1.
- 1250mg/m^2 on day 1 and 8 of a 21-day treatment cycle in combination with paclitaxel 175mg/m^2.

♣ Dose adjustments

Myelosuppression

- ↓ to 75% of the original dose in event of:
  - absolute granulocyte count < 500 × 10^6/L for >5 days
  - absolute granulocyte count < 100 × 10^6/L for >3 days
  - febrile neutropenia
  - platelets < 25,000 × 10^6/L
  - delay in cycle of > 1 week due to toxicity.
- Dose modifications within cycle are summarized in the manufacturer's Summary of Product Characteristics (SPC).

Hepatic/renal impairment

- Caution should be exercised in patients with hepatic or renal insufficiency (GFR <30ml/min), though there are insufficient data to guide dosing recommendations.

☞ Pharmacology

Gemcitabine is a pyrimidine analogue, which is converted to the active forms gemcitabine diphosphate, (dFdCDP) and gemcitabine triphosphate (dFdCTP) intracellularly. dFdCDP inhibits ribonuclease reductase and thus reduces the intracellular pool of deoxyribonucleotide triphosphates (dNTPs). Additionally, dFdCTP competes with dCTP for incorporation into DNA. Both contribute to inhibition of DNA synthesis. Gemcitabine and its metabolites are renally excreted, though pharmacokinetics are unaffected by mild to moderate renal insufficiency (GFR 30–80ml/min).

Goserelin acetate

Zoladex®, Novgos® (POM)
- Implant in pre-filled syringes 3.6mg, 10.6mg.

Indications
- Prostate cancer: metastatic, locally advanced prostate cancer. As an adjuvant treatment to radiotherapy in patients with high-risk localized or locally advanced prostate cancer. As neoadjuvant treatment prior to radiotherapy in patients with high-risk localized or locally advanced prostate cancer. As adjuvant treatment to radical prostatectomy in patients with locally advanced prostate cancer at high risk of disease progression
- Advanced breast cancer in pre- and perimenopausal women suitable for hormonal manipulation. Indicated as an alternative to chemotherapy in the standard of care for pre/perimenopausal women with oestrogen receptor-positive early breast cancer.
- Also used in benign conditions and for assisted reproduction.

Contraindications and precautions
- Hypersensitivity to the active substance or any of the excipients is a contraindication.

☺ Undesirable effects
Common
- Erectile dysfunction
- Hot flush
- Hyperhidrosis
- ↓ libido.

Uncommon
- Blood pressure abnormal
- Bone density ↓
- Bone pain
- Cardiac failure
- Drug hypersensitivity
- Glucose intolerance
- Gynaecomastia
- Injection site reaction
- Mood changes and depression
- Myocardial infarction
- Rash
- Weight ↑.

Rare
- Anaphylactic reaction
- Arthralgia
- Breast tenderness
- Pituitary haemorrhage
- Psychotic disorders.

Drug interactions
Pharmacokinetic
- None known.

Pharmacodynamic
- None known.

♨ Dose
- For prostate and breast cancer 3.6mg is implanted subcutaneously into the anterior abdominal wall every 28 days. 3-monthly preparations can also be used as an alternative to monthly.

♂ Dose adjustments
● No dose adjustments necessary.

Additional information
● For men with prostate cancer testosterone levels can be measured to monitor the effectiveness of goserelin.

⟩ Pharmacology
Goserelin is a synthetic analogue of naturally occurring LHRH. With continued use it results in inhibition of pituitary luteinizing hormone (LH) secretion leading to a fall in serum testosterone concentrations in males and serum oestradiol concentrations in females. This effect is reversible on discontinuation of therapy. Along with other LHRH agonists goserelin, when first used, may transiently increase serum testosterone concentration in men, and serum oestradiol concentration in women. In men at risk of spinal cord compression or ureteric obstruction, initial use may potentiate these complications unless an androgen antagonist is used as protective cover.

Hexamethylmelamine

Altretamine/Hexalen® (POM)
- Capsules: 50mg.

Indications
- Relapsed or treatment refractory ovarian cancer.

Contraindications and precautions
- Patients should be given prophylactic antiemetics.
- If neurological symptoms fail to stabilize on reduced dose schedules, capsules should be discontinued.

☺ Undesirable effects
Common
- Abdominal pain
- Anorexia
- Depression
- Dizziness
- Fatigue
- Mood changes
- Myelosuppression
- Nausea
- Peripheral neuropathy
- Vomiting.

Uncommon
- Abdominal pain.

Rare
- Alopecia
- Hepatic toxicity
- Pruritus
- Rash.

Drug interactions
Pharmacokinetic
- Concurrent administration of monoamine oxidase (MAO) antidepressants may cause severe orthostatic hypotension.

Pharmacodynamic
- When used with other neurotoxic agents the risk of neurotoxicity is ↑.

♣ Dose
- Oral monotherapy 260mg/m^2/day for 14–21 days every 28 days. Total daily dose given as 4 divided oral doses.

♣ Dose adjustments
- Dose interruptions required for neutropenia <1.0 × 10^9/L or thrombocytopenia <75 × 10^9/L; progressive neurotoxicity or GI intolerance unresponsive to symptomatic measures. Subsequently restart at 200mg/m^2 per day.

Additional information
- Capsules should be taken after meals, and should be swallowed whole.
- Neurological examination should be performed regularly, and peripheral blood counts at least monthly.

✧ Pharmacology

Hexamethylmelamine is thought to act as an alkylating agent. It is well absorbed following oral administration but is rapidly and extensively demethylated in the liver. The principal metabolites are pentamethyl-melamine and tetramethylmelamine. Peak plasma levels generally occur at between 0.5 and 3 hours after administration.

Hydroxycarbamide

Hydrea® (POM)
- Capsules: 500mg.

Indications
- Treatment of CML.
- Essential thrombocythaemia or primary polycythaemia with a high risk of thromboembolism.
- Treatment of carcinoma of the cervix in conjunction with radiotherapy.

Contraindications and precautions
- May be mutagenic so patients advised to use reliable contraception during, and for a minimum of 3 months after, taking the drug.

☺ Undesirable effects
Common
- Diarrhoea or constipation
- Leucopenia
- Raised mean corpuscular volume.

Uncommon
- Anaemia, thrombocytopenia
- Mucositis
- Rash
- Vomiting.

Rare
- Leg ulcers which can be difficult to treat
- Second malignancy.

Drug interactions
Pharmacokinetic
- Hydroxycarbamide does not interact widely with other drugs.

Pharmacodynamic
- Clozapine: increases risk of agranulocytosis.

♣ Dose
- CML: 20–30mg/kg OD, continuous.
- Polycythaemia/ET: 15–20mg/kg starting dose OD, continuous.

♣ Dose adjustments
- Use with caution in severe renal dysfunction.

♦ Pharmacology
Interferes with synthesis of DNA through poorly defined mechanisms.

Idarubicin

Zavedos® (POM)

- 5mg or 10mg capsules, for oral use.
- 5mg or 10mg vials, powder for reconstitution, for IV use.

Indications

- AML (often in combination with other agents such as fludarabine and cytarabine).
- Advanced breast cancer as a single agent, after treatment failed with first-line chemotherapy not including anthracyclines.

Contraindications and precautions

- Patients with severe cardiac dysfunction, recent myocardial infarction, or severe arrhythmia.
- Severe hepatic or renal dysfunction.
- Use with caution in patients previously treated with anthracycline and/or anthracenediones—monitor cumulative doses.
- Fertility:
  - Advise barrier contraception during and for 3 months after therapy.
  - Risk of sterility—advise sperm storage for men.

☹ Undesirable effects

Common

- Alopecia
- Asymptomatic reduction in left ventricular function
- Elevation of liver enzymes/bilirubin (usually transient)
- Mucositis
- Myelosuppression
- Nausea
- Rash
- Red colouration of urine for 1–2 days post infusion
- Tachyarrhythmias.

Uncommon

- Acute arrhythmia
- Cardiomyopathy with cardiac failure
- Oesophagitis, erosive gastritis.

Rare

- Acral erythema
- Secondary leukaemia.

Drug interactions

Pharmacokinetic

- Idarubicin does not interact with many other drugs.

Pharmacodynamic

- Myelosuppressive effect potentiated by other myelosuppressive drugs.
- Associated mucositis may interfere with absorption of concurrently used oral medications.
- May exacerbate cardiotoxicity of other drugs which can cause this side effect.

Dose
- Regimen specific.
- Typical dose when used in AML in combination with fludarabine and cytarabine (so-called FLA-Ida) is 8mg/m^2 daily IV for 3 consecutive doses.

Dose adjustments
- Doses should be reduced in the setting of raised creatinine or raised bilirubin.
- Avoid using in severe renal and/or hepatic impairment.
  Typical modification is to reduce dose by 50% when creatinine 100–175micromol/L, and by 50% when bilirubin 40–85micromol/L.

Additional information
- The maximum cumulative dose for idarubicin is considered to be 400mg/m^2.

Pharmacology
Intercalates with DNA preventing action of topoisomerase II and therefore inhibiting DNA replication. Highly lipophilic molecule resulting in more rapid cellular uptake than both doxorubicin and daunorubicin. Shown to have a higher potency than these 2 agents, and has an improved therapeutic index with respect to cardiotoxicity.

Ifosfamide

Ifex®, Mitoxana® (POM)

- Solution for injection/infusion: 1g/25ml, 2g/50ml.

Indications

- Ewing's sarcoma
- Osteosarcoma
- STS
- Relapsed testicular seminoma and NSGCT.

Contraindications

- History of hypersensitivity to ifosfamide
- Inflammation of urinary bladder
- Renal or hepatic impairment
- Pregnancy and lactation.

Precautions

- ↑ risk of cardiotoxicity with:
  - previous anthracycline therapy
  - inclusion of heart in previous radiotherapy fields.
- ↑ risk of encephalopathy with:
  - impaired renal function
  - previous nephrotoxic drugs
  - general debility/advanced age.
- ► Encephalopathy may be reversed by administration of methylene blue 50mg of a 1–2% TDS/4 times daily (QDS).
- ► Concurrent administration of mesna is required to reduce incidence of haemorrhagic cystitis (see 📖 Dose, p.168).
- Fertility:
  - Advise barrier contraception during and for 3 months after therapy.
  - Risk of sterility—advise sperm storage for men.

☺ Undesirable effects

Common

- Nausea and vomiting (moderate emetic risk)
- Alopecia
- Encephalopathy/drowsiness
- Microscopic haematuria
- Nephrotoxicity including ↓GFR and tubular dysfunction (may be dose-limiting at high doses)
- Myelosuppression (nadir 7–10 days post therapy).

Uncommon

- Acute and chronic renal failure
- Aminoaciduria/phosphaturia
- Syndrome of inappropriate antidiuretic hormone secretion (SIADH).

Rare

- Cardiotoxicity (at high doses)
- Radiation recall

- Renal Fanconi syndrome
- Second malignancies.

Drug interactions
- Cytochrome P450 inducers/inhibitors: avoid if possible
- Nephrotoxic drugs: ↑ risk of nephrotoxicity and neurotoxicity
- Sulphonylureas: ↑ hypoglycaemic action
- Warfarin: ↑ anticoagulant effect.

Dose
Fractionated
- 8–12g/m^2 fractionated as single daily doses over 3–5 days every 2–4 weeks.

As continuous infusion
- 5–6g/m^2 (maximum 10g) as 24-hour infusion every 2–4 weeks.

Concurrent mesna
- Ifosfamide must be given with mesna to minimize risk of haemorrhagic cystitis
- See p.168 for details on mesna dosing.

Dose adjustments
For toxicity
- Consider dose reduction for significant myelosuppression.

General
- Consideration of elective dose reduction should be made in elderly patients.

⊘ Pharmacology
Ifosfamide is an analogue of cyclophosphamide that mediates cytotoxic effect by alkylation of DNA. Following administration, ifosfamide is hydroxylated by CYP3A4 to the active 4-hydroxy-ifosfamide and subsequently metabolized to active aldoifosfamide. The chloroacetaldehyde metabolite of ifosfamide is believed responsible for neurotoxic effects. Both ifosfamide and its metabolites are renally excreted; following single dose 80% dose is eliminated by 72 hours. Excretion is delayed in presence of renal impairment.

Imatinib

Glivec® (POM)
- Tablet: 100mg (scored—60); 400mg (30).

Indications
- ALL
- Advanced hypereosinophilic syndrome and chronic eosinophilic leukaemia
- CML (accelerated and chronic phase; blast crisis)
- Dermatofibrosarcoma protuberans
- Gastrointestinal stromal tumours (GISTs)
- Myelodysplastic/myeloproliferative diseases.

Contraindications and precautions
- Use cautiously in the following:
  - cardiac disease (risk of fluid retention and subsequent cardiac failure)
  - concomitant use with drugs that inhibit CYP3A4
  - diabetes (can cause hyperglycaemia)
  - elderly
  - gout (can cause hyperuricaemia)
  - hepatic impairment
  - renal impairment.
- Patients should ideally not use high doses of paracetamol with imatinib since glucuronidation may be affected.
- Imatinib may cause dizziness and fatigue. Patients should be advised to not drive (or operate machinery) if affected.

Adverse effects
Very common
- Abdominal pain
- Anaemia
- Arthralgia
- Bone pain
- Dermatitis/eczema/rash
- Diarrhoea
- Dyspepsia
- Fatigue
- Fluid retention
- Headache
- Muscle spasm and cramps
- Myalgia
- Nausea
- Neutropenia
- Periorbital oedema
- Thrombocytopenia
- Vomiting
- Weight increase (likely fluid retention).

Common
- Anorexia
- Blurred vision
- Conjunctival haemorrhage
- Conjunctivitis
- Constipation
- Cough
- Dizziness
- Dry eye
- Dry mouth
- Dyspnoea
- Epistaxis
- Eyelid oedema
- Febrile neutropenia
- Flatulence
- Flushing
- Gastritis
- Gastro-oesophageal reflux
- Hypoaesthesia

- Insomnia
- Lacrimation ↑
- Night sweats
- Pancytopenia
- Paraesthesia
- Photosensitivity reaction

- Pruritus
- Pyrexia
- Raised LFTs
- Taste disturbance
- Weight loss.

Uncommon

- Acute renal failure
- Gastric ulcer
- Gout/hyperuricaemia
- Haematuria
- Hepatitis
- Hypercalcaemia
- Hyperglycaemia

- Hypertension
- Hypokalaemia
- Jaundice
- Oesophagitis
- Pleural effusion
- Sexual dysfunction
- Stomatitis.

Drug interactions

Pharmacokinetic

- Imatinib is metabolized by CYP3A4; it is also an inhibitor of CYP3A4 and possibly CYP2C9. Co-administration with drugs that are metabolized by, or affect the activity of this pathway may lead to clinically relevant drug interactions and the prescriber should be aware that dosage adjustments may be necessary, particularly of drugs with a narrow therapeutic index.
- Paracetamol—glucuronidation inhibited by imatinib; potential paracetamol toxicity with prolonged use.
- Warfarin—manufacturer advises use of low-molecular-weight heparin with imatinib.
- Avoid grapefruit juice as it may increase the bioavailability of imatinib through inhibition of intestinal CYP3A4.

Pharmacodynamic

- None known.

⚖ Dose

Acute lymphoblastic leukaemia

- 600mg PO OD.

Advanced hypereosinophilic syndrome and chronic eosinophilic leukaemia

- 600mg PO OD, ↑ if necessary to max. dose of 400mg PO BD.

Chronic myeloid leukaemia

- Accelerated phase: 600mg PO OD, ↑ if necessary to max. dose 400mg PO BD.
- Blast crisis: 600mg PO OD, ↑ if necessary to max. dose 400mg PO BD.
- Chronic phase: 400mg PO OD, ↑ if necessary to max. dose 400mg PO BD.

Dermatofibrosarcoma protuberans

- 400mg PO BD.

GISTs
- 400mg PO OD.

Myelodysplastic/myeloproliferative diseases
- 400mg PO OD.

> **♣️ Dose adjustments for adverse reactions**
> - If severe non-haematological adverse effects occur, imatinib should
>   be discontinued until the event has resolved. Imatinib can be
>   re-introduced as appropriate at a reduced dose:
>   - 400mg PO OD: reduce dose to 300mg PO OD
>   - 600mg PO OD: reduce dose to 400mg PO OD
>   - 400mg PO BD: reduce dose to 600mg PO OD.
> - Refer to the SPC if haematological adverse effects occur.

♣️ Dose adjustments

Elderly
- No dose adjustments are necessary.

Hepatic/renal impairment
- Imatinib is significantly metabolized by the liver. Patients with mild,
  moderate, or severe liver impairment should be given the minimum
  recommended dose of 400mg PO OD. The dose can be reduced if not
  tolerated.
- For patients with renal impairment (CrCl <60ml/min) or those on
  dialysis, the recommended maximum starting dose is 400mg PO OD.

Additional information
- Tablets should be taken with a meal and a large glass of water to
  minimize the risk of GI irritation.
- If necessary, tablets may be dispersed in water or apple juice (~50ml
  for a 100mg tablet, and 200ml for a 400mg tablet) immediately prior to
  administration.

⊸ Pharmacology

Imatinib is a Bcr-Abl tyrosine kinase inhibitor which is the product of the
Philadelphia chromosome in CML. It induces apoptosis in Bcr-Abl-positive
cell lines as well as in fresh leukaemic cells in Philadelphia chromosome-
positive CML. It also inhibits other tyrosine kinases and inhibits proliferation and induces apoptosis in GIST cells. It is well absorbed after oral
administration, with a bioavailability of 98% and is highly protein bound. It
is extensively metabolized, mainly by CYP3A4, to a compound with similar
activity. Imatinib and its metabolites are not excreted via the kidney to a
significant extent.

Interferon alfa

Roferon-A® (POM) (interferon alfa-2a)
- Pre-filled syringes with solution: 3MIU, 4.5MIU, 6MIU, 9MIU (MIU = million international units).

Intron-A® (POM) (interferon alfa-2b)
- Solution vials for injection: 18MIU, 25MIU
- Prefilled multidose pens for injection: 3MIU, 5MIU, 10MIU

Sylatron™ (POM) (pegylated interferon alfa-2b)
- Lyophilized powder per single-use vial: 296mcg, 444mcg, 888mcg.

Indications
- Malignant melanoma: as adjuvant therapy post-resection of stage II disease (only approved indication for Sylatron™).
- Metastatic renal cell carcinoma.
- Hairy cell leukaemia.
- Cutaneous T-cell lymphoma.
- Follicular non-Hodgkin lymphoma: as an adjunct to chemotherapy.
- CML (Philadelphia chromosome-positive, chronic phase): either as monotherapy or in combination with cytarabine (Ara-C).
- Multiple myeloma: as maintenance therapy following initial induction chemotherapy.

Contraindications and precautions
- Contraindicated if pre-existing severe cardiac, renal, hepatic, or myeloid dysfunction, significant cardiac history, and in chronic hepatitis patients recently treated with immunosuppressive agents.
- Use with caution in transplant patients, in patients with diabetes (anti-diabetic regimen may need adjusting) and in patients predisposed to autoimmune diseases.

☹ Undesirable effects
Common
- Abdominal pain
- Anorexia
- Arrhythmias
- Arthralgia
- Chest pain
- Diarrhoea
- Fatigue
- Fever
- Flu-like symptoms
- Myalgia
- Myelosuppression
- Nausea
- Oedema
- Palpitations
- Vomiting.

Uncommon
- Alopecia
- Confusion
- Depression
- Dizziness
- Hypertension
- Hypotension
- Paraesthesia
- Reduced fertility
- Suicidal ideation
- Visual disturbance.

Rare
- Haemolytic anaemia
- Hyperglycaemia
- Infection
- Pulmonary/renal/hepatic dysfunction
- Thyroid dysfunction.

Drug interactions

Pharmacokinetic
- Interferon alfa reportedly reduces the clearance of theophylline.

Pharmacodynamic
- The neurotoxic, haematotoxic, or cardiotoxic effects of other drugs may be ↑ by interferons.
- Pulmonary dysfunction is reported more frequently when interferon-alfa is taken concomitantly with shosaikoto (a Chinese herbal medicine).

♏ Dose
- Melanoma:
  - Induction therapy: Intron-A® 20MIU/m^2 IV daily 5 days a week for 4 weeks (monitor FBC and LFTs weekly)
  - Maintenance therapy: Intron-A® 10 MIU/m^2 SC 3 times a week for 48 weeks (monitor FBC and LFTs monthly)
- CML: 4–5MIU/m^2 SC daily
- Other indications: 3–18MIU SC 3 times a week for 3–18 months
- (Peginterferon in melanoma: 6mcg/kg per week SC for 8 doses, then 3mcg/kg per week SC for up to 5 years.)

♏ Dose adjustments
- If neutrophils <0.5 × 10^9/L or ALT/AST >5 × ULN or intolerable toxicity, interrupt therapy until toxicity resolves, then restart with a 50% dose reduction.
- If neutrophils <0.25 × 10^9/L or ALT/AST >10 × ULN or intolerable toxicity occurs despite dose reduction, stop interferon therapy.
- If pulmonary symptoms develop, stop interferon and start corticosteroids.

Additional information
- Store at 2–8°C (peginterferon: 15–30°C). Do not freeze.

⌖ Pharmacology
Interferons are cytokines, which play various roles in the immune system, including activating NK cells and macrophages, upregulating antigen presentation, and impairing viral replication within host cells. The mechanisms by which interferons exert antitumour activity are not fully known, but are thought to include modulating the immune system as well as reducing DNA, RNA, and protein synthesis. Following SC injection, C$_{max}$ is reached within 3–12 hours. Interferon alfa is eliminated renally.

Interleukin-2 (Aldesleukin)

Proleukin® (POM)

- Powder for solution for injection/infusion: 18×10^6IU.

Indications

- Metastatic renal cell carcinoma.

Contraindications and precautions

- Contraindicated if:
  - ECOG (Eastern Cooperative Oncology Group) performance status ≥2.
  - ECOG performance status ≥1 *and* >1 organ with metastatic disease *and* <24 months between initial diagnosis of primary tumour being considered for interleukin-2 (IL-2) therapy.
  - pre-existing auto-immune disease, significant cardiac disease, organ allografts, active infection requiring antibiotics or active CNS metastases.
  - white blood cell (WBC) $<4.0 \times 10^9$/L, platelets $<100 \times 10^9$/L, haematocrit <30%, elevated bilirubin or creatinine outside normal range.
- Use with caution in elderly patients, as they may be more susceptible to side effects.
- Treatment with IL-2 can worsen effusions from serosal surfaces (e.g. pericardial effusions), so consider draining these prior to starting IL-2 therapy.

☺ Undesirable effects

Common
- Anorexia
- Capillary leak syndrome
- Fatigue
- Flu-like symptoms
- ↑ risk of infection
- Myelosuppression
- Nausea/vomiting/diarrhoea
- Rash/pruritus.

Uncommon
- Confusion/depression/somnolence
- Convulsions/paralysis
- Cough/dyspnoea
- Impaired kidney function
- Myocardial infarction/cardiovascular disorders
- Vitiligo.

Rare
- Alopecia
- Cerebral vasculitis
- PE
- Stevens–Johnson syndrome.

Drug interactions

Pharmacokinetic
- No specific pharmacokinetic interactions have been reported.

Pharmacodynamic
- Concomitant treatment with cisplatin, vinblastine, or dacarbazine is not recommended due to incidents of fatal tumour lysis syndrome.
- Concomitant treatment with steroids may reduce the activity of IL-2 and so should be avoided, unless they are being used to treat IL-2-induced severe immune toxicity.
- Contrast media should be avoided within 2 weeks after any IL-2 therapy, due to risk of toxicity.

Dose
- Week 1: 18×10^6IU injection SC daily for 5 days, then rest for 2 days.
- Weeks 2–4: 18×10^6IU injection SC days 1 & 2, then 9×10^6IU days 3–5, then rest for 2 days.
- 1 week rest, then repeat.

Dose adjustments
- If intolerable toxicity develops, the dose should be reduced or treatment interrupted until the toxicity has settled.
- Treatment should be discontinued in patients who develop severe lethargy or somnolence, due to risk of coma.

Additional information
- Store at 2–8°C. Do not freeze.

Pharmacology
IL-2 is a naturally occurring cytokine that stimulates the immune system by increasing the growth and activity of both B and T lymphocytes. IL-2 produced in the laboratory is called aldesleukin. If administered as a short IV bolus, the serum half-life is bi-exponential, with a half-life in the α-phase of 13min and in the -phase of 85min. If administered subcutaneously, the half-life is longer at 3–5 hours. Aldesleukin is mainly metabolized and cleared by the kidneys.

Ipilimumab

Yervoy™ (POM)

- 5mg/ml concentrate for solution for infusion.

Indications

- Treatment of advanced (unresectable or metastatic) melanoma in adults who have received prior therapy (at 3mg/kg dose).

Contraindications and precautions

- Ipilimumab should be avoided in patients with severe active autoimmune disease or ↑ risk of graft rejection, where further immune activation could be potentially life threatening.
- Ipilimumab should be used with caution in other patients with a history of autoimmune disease.

☺ Undesirable effects

Common

- Anaemia
- Constipation
- Cough/dyspnoea
- Diarrhoea/colitis
- Fatigue
- Fever
- Headache
- Nausea/vomiting/anorexia
- Peripheral sensory neuropathy
- Pruritus/rash/dermatitis
- Tumour-related pain.

Uncommon

- Colitis/enterocolitis
- Hepatotoxicity
- Hypopituitarism/hypothyroidism/adrenal insufficiency
- Intestinal perforation
- Nephritis
- Stevens–Johnson syndrome/toxic epidermal necrolysis.

Rare

- Acute respiratory distress syndrome/pneumonitis
- Angiopathy/vasculitis
- Guillain–Barré syndrome
- Haemolytic anaemia
- Meningism
- Pancreatitis
- Pericarditis.

Drug interactions

Pharmacokinetic

- Ipilimumab does not interact significantly with other medications.

Pharmacodynamic

- Avoid using systemic corticosteroids before starting a course of ipilimumab as this may reduce treatment efficacy.
- The use of systemic corticosteroids during ipilimumab therapy, to treat immune-related adverse reactions, does not appear to impair treatment efficacy.

.ṣ Dose

- Current licensed indication is 3mg/kg administered IV over 90min every 3 weeks for a total of 4 doses.
- Treatment with 10mg/kg is currently being investigated in clinical trials.

.ṣ Dose adjustments

- Dose reductions are not recommended. Doses that are omitted due to adverse reactions must not be replaced.
- Omit scheduled dose of ipilimumab if patient develops:
  - grade 2 diarrhoea or neuropathy
  - grade 3 rash or hepatotoxicity (AST/ALT ≥5 × ULN or total bilirubin ≥ 3 × ULN)
  - severe endocrinopathy that is not controlled with hormone replacement therapy or high-dose immunosuppressive therapy.
- Permanently discontinue ipilimumab if patient develops:
  - grade 3 or 4 diarrhoea or colitis
  - grade 3 or 4 neuropathy
  - grade 4 rash
  - AST/ALT > 8 × ULN or total bilirubin > 5 × ULN.
- Patients with grade 3 or 4 endocrinopathy controlled with hormone replacement therapy may remain on therapy.

Additional information

- Immune-related adverse reactions can develop months after the last dose of ipilimumab has been administered.
- Early diagnosis and appropriate management of immune-related adverse reactions are essential to minimize life-threatening complications.
- Severe immune-related adverse reactions should be treated with systemic high-dose corticosteroids with or without additional immunosuppressive therapy (e.g. infliximab 5mg/kg).
- High-dose corticosteroid therapy should be tapered down gradually (over at least 1 month).

⊹ Pharmacology

Ipilimumab is a fully humanized monoclonal antibody against cytotoxic T-lymphocyte antigen-4 (CTLA-4). CTLA-4 is a negative regulator of T-cell activation. By blocking the inhibitory signal of CTLA-4, ipilimumab potentiates T-cell activation, proliferation, and lymphocyte infiltration into tumours, leading to tumour cell death.

Irinotecan

Campto® (POM)

- Irinotecan 20mg/ml, concentrate for solution for infusion. Clear yellow solution.

Indications

Irinotecan is indicated for the treatment of patients with advanced or metastatic colorectal cancer.

- In combination with 5-FU/folinic acid (plus or minus bevacizumab) in patients in first-line therapy.
- As a single agent in patients in second-line therapy.
- In combination with cetuximab in patients with EGFR-expressing, KRAS wild-type metastatic colorectal cancer, who had not received prior treatment for metastatic disease or after failure of irinotecan-including cytotoxic therapy
- In combination with capecitabine but extreme caution is required due to the overlapping toxicities of both neutropenia and diarrhoea.

Contraindications and precautions

Contraindications

- Chronic inflammatory bowel disease and/or bowel obstruction.
- History of severe hypersensitivity reactions to irinotecan hydrochloride trihydrate or to any of the excipients.
- Pregnancy and lactation.
- Bilirubin >3× ULN.
- Severe bone marrow failure.
- World Health Organization performance status >2.
- Concomitant use with St John's wort.

Cautions

- An ↑ risk of diarrhoea is seen in those who have had previous abdominal/pelvic radiotherapy. If not appropriately treated, the diarrhoea can be life threatening, especially if the patient is concomitantly neutropenic.
- Hepatic impairment: in patients with bilirubin levels of 1.5–3× ULN, the single agent recommended dose of irinotecan is 200mg/m^2. Although no specific recommended dose is given for irinotecan given in combination when there is hepatic impairment, it is sensible to consider a reduction of 40%. Patients with bilirubin levels above 3× the ULN, should not be treated with irinotecan.
- Renal impairment: no data exist in renal impairment and irinotecan should be used with caution. One small study suggested an ↑ risk of neutropenia.

☺ Undesirable effects

Common

- Acute cholinergic syndrome (treatable with atropine)
- Anaemia, neutropenia, thrombocytopenia, lymphopenia
- Fatigue, alopecia
- Febrile neutropenia (more common with single-agent 3-weekly use)
- Hepatic enzyme increases
- Nausea, vomiting, abdominal pain, and severe delayed diarrhoea.

Uncommon
- Interstitial lung disease
- Intestinal obstruction, ileus, or GI haemorrhage
- Pseudomembranous colitis
- Renal insufficiency, hypotension or cardio-circulatory failure as a consequence of dehydration associated with diarrhoea and/or vomiting.

Rare
- Hypokalaemia, hyponatraemia
- Intestinal perforation.

Drug interactions
Pharmacokinetic
- Metabolized by CYP3A4 and can be affected by co-administration of other inhibitors or inducers of CYP3A4.

Pharmacodynamic
- In combination studies with bevacizumab, there is an ↑ risk of diarrhoea compared to cytotoxic(s) alone.

,ᴊ Dose
- Single agent: 350mg/m^2 as an infusion over 30–90min every 3 weeks.
- In combination with 5-FU: 180mg/m^2 as an infusion over 30–90min every 2 weeks.

,ᴊ Dose adjustments
With the following adverse events a dose reduction of 15–20% should be applied for irinotecan (and 5-FU when applicable):
- For haematological toxicity: neutropenia grade 4, febrile neutropenia (neutropenia grade 3–4 and fever grade 2–4), thrombocytopenia and leucopenia (grade 4)
- Non-haematological toxicity: grade 3–4.

Additional information
- As irinotecan can occasionally cause impairment of the hepatic enzymes, this can be confused with disease progression. Interpret with care.

⊕ Pharmacology
Irinotecan is a semisynthetic derivative of the plant alkaloid camptothecin, and is bioactivated by carboxylesterases to the topoisomerase I inhibitor SN-38, a minor metabolite predominantly in the liver. Intestinal carboxylesterases can also generate SN-38, followed by subsequent oral absorption. A second major polar metabolite of irinotecan, aminopentanecarboxylic acid (APC), is the product of CYP3A4-mediated oxidation. APC is 100× less active than SN-38 as a topoisomerase I inhibitor. SN-38 is eliminated mainly through conjugation by hepatic uridine glucuronosyltransferase (UGT1.1), the same isoezyme responsible for glucuronidation of bilirubin. Grade 4 irinotecan-related toxicity (i.e. neutropenia, diarrhoea) has been reported in patients with deficient UGT1.1 activity (Gilbert's syndrome), so caution if there is a clinical suspicion or definitive proof of the presence of this syndrome.

Lapatinib

Tyverb® (POM)

- 250mg film-coated tablets.

Indications

- Breast cancer overexpressing HER2:
  - With capecitabine in metastatic disease progressing after treatment including anthracyclines, a taxane, and trastuzumab.
  - With an aromatase inhibitor in patients with metastatic hormone receptor-positive disease not intending for chemotherapy.

Contraindications and precautions

- Patients with pre-existing left ventricular dysfunction should not be treated with lapatinib.
- Left ventricular function should be monitored on treatment.

☺ Undesirable effects

Very common

- Alopecia
- Arthralgia
- Cough
- Diarrhoea
- Dyspnoea
- Fatigue
- Headache
- Insomnia
- Nausea
- Rash.

Common

- Constipation
- Dehydration
- Hepatotoxicity
- Left ventricular dysfunction
- Nail disorders.

Uncommon and rare side effects include:

- Anaphylaxis
- Pneumonitis.

Drug interactions

Pharmacokinetic

- Potent inhibitors or inducers of cytochrome P450 enzyme CYP3A4 affect the AUC of lapatinib.
- Lapatinib inhibits cytochrome P450 enzyme CYP2C8.
- Caution should be used when dosing lapatinib with medications with narrow therapeutic windows that are substrates of P-gp such as digoxin.

⚡ Dose

- With capecitabine: 1250mg PO OD.
- With aromatase inhibitors: 1500mg PO OD.

⚡ Dose adjustments

- Dosing should be interrupted for persistent grade 2 toxicities, and resumed at full dose or with a decrease of 250mg/day once these have resolved to grade 1 or better.

- Lapatinib should be discontinued if left ventricular dysfunction or pneumonitis develop.

⊕ Pharmacology

Lapatinib is a protein tyrosine kinase inhibitor and inhibits ErbB-driven tumour cell growth. It targets the intracellular tyrosine kinase domains of both the EGFR (ErbB1) and of HER2 (ErbB2) receptors.

Letrozole

Femara® (POM)

- Tablet: 2.5mg (14; 28).

Indications

- Treatment (primary or adjuvant) of postmenopausal women with hormone receptor-positive invasive early breast cancer.

Contraindications and precautions

- Letrozole is contraindicated for use in patients with:
  - severe hepatic impairment
  - unknown or negative receptor status.
- It should be used with caution in patients with severe renal impairment (CrCl <10ml/min).
- May cause reduction in bone mineral density; treatment for osteoporosis may be required.
- Fatigue and dizziness have been reported with letrozole. Caution should be observed when driving or operating machinery while such symptoms persist.

Adverse effects

Very common

- Arthralgia
- Hot flushes.

Common

- Alopecia
- Anorexia
- Bone fractures
- Bone pain
- Constipation
- Depression
- Diarrhoea
- Dizziness
- Dyspepsia
- Fatigue
- Headache
- Myalgia
- Osteoporosis
- Nausea
- Peripheral oedema
- Raised serum cholesterol
- Sweating
- Vomiting.

Uncommon

- Anxiety
- Drowsiness
- Dyspnoea
- Hypertension
- Ischaemic cardiac events
- Leucopenia
- Tumour pain
- Urinary tract infection
- Vaginal bleeding/discharge
- Visual disturbances.

Drug interactions

Pharmacokinetic

- Letrozole is metabolized by CYP2A6 and CYP3A4; it inhibits CYP2A6 and also moderately affects CYP2C19. Co-administration with drugs that are metabolized by, or affect the activity of these pathways may lead to clinically relevant drug interactions and the prescriber should be aware that dosage adjustments may be necessary, particularly of drugs with a narrow therapeutic index.

LETROZOLE **151**

- Letrozole is unlikely to be a cause of many drug interactions since CYP2A6 does not have a major role in drug metabolism. At usual doses, letrozole is unlikely to affect CYP2C19 substrates.

Pharmacodynamic
- None known.

⚬ Dose
- 2.5mg PO OD.

⚬ Dose adjustments
Elderly
- No dose adjustments are necessary for elderly patients.

Hepatic/renal impairment
- No dose adjustments are necessary for patients with mild–moderate hepatic impairment or mild–moderate renal impairment (CrCl ≥10ml/min).
- Letrozole is contraindicated for use in severe hepatic impairment and should be used with caution in severe renal impairment (due to lack of data).

Additional information
- Letrozole should be continued for 5 years or until tumour relapse occurs.

⟐ Pharmacology
Letrozole is a non-steroidal aromatase inhibitor. It is believed to work by significantly lowering serum oestradiol concentrations through inhibition of aromatase (converts adrenal androstenedione to oestrone, which is precursor of oestradiol). Many breast cancers have oestrogen receptors and growth of these tumours can be stimulated by oestrogens.

Leuprorelin acetate

Prostap® SR (POM)

- 3.75mg, powder and solvent for solution for injection.

Eligard® (POM)

- 22.5mg, powder and solvent for solution for injection.

Indications

- Hormone-dependent locally advanced and metastatic prostate cancer.
- As adjuvant treatment following radiotherapy or radical prostatectomy in patients with high-risk localized or locally advanced prostate cancer.

Contraindications and precautions

- Contraindicated in patients who have already undergone surgical castration (leuprorelin will not further decrease testosterone levels).
- Contraindicated as monotherapy in patients with spinal metastases or spinal cord compression due to risk of tumour flare.
- Should be used with caution in patients with ↑ risk of osteoporosis.

☹ Undesirable effects

Common

- Arthralgia/myalgia
- Bone demineralization (proportional to time on treatment)
- Bruising/erythema/pruritus
- Fatigue
- Gynaecomastia/breast tenderness
- Hot flushes
- Nausea/diarrhoea
- Reduced libido
- Weight gain.

Uncommon

- Altered taste/sense of smell
- Changes in glucose tolerance
- Depression
- Dry mouth
- Headache
- Hypertension.

Rare

- Abnormal involuntary movements
- Alopecia
- Flatulence
- Hepatic dysfunction
- Pituitary apoplexy
- Syncope
- Thrombocytopenia/leucopenia
- Thromboembolic events.

Drug interactions

Pharmacokinetic

- No specific pharmacokinetic interactions have been reported.

Pharmacodynamic

- No specific pharmacodynamic interactions have been reported.

⚗ Dose

- Prostap®: 3.75mg injection SC or IM every month.
- Eligard®: 22.5mg injection SC every 3 months.

♣ Dose adjustments

• To continue on treatment as long as patient is tolerating and disease is under control.

Additional information

• Testosterone levels can initially rise during first 3–4 days on treatment.
• Antiandrogen cover starting 3 days prior to leuprolide therapy and continuing for first 2–3 weeks of treatment can prevent initial tumour flare.
• As with other SC medications the injection site should be varied periodically.

♦ Pharmacology

Leuprorelin acetate is a synthetic analogue of GnRH. The drug comes as a pre-filled syringe of powder, along with a second pre-filled syringe of solvent. The 2 are mixed together to form a single solution that is then injected subcutaneously. The injected solution forms a solid medicinal product, which provides continuous release of leuprorelin over a 3-month period. Leuprorelin treatment initially increases circulating levels of LH and follicle stimulating hormone (FSH), leading to a transient rise in testosterone. Continuing treatment with leuprorelin inhibits LH/FSH secretion and so decreases testosterone production, usually after 3–5 weeks of therapy. Long-term studies have demonstrated testosterone suppression lasting up to 7 years.

Liposomal doxorubicin

Caelyx® (POM)
- 2mg/ml concentrate for infusion.

Myocet® (POM)
- 50mg powder and pre-admixtures for concentrate for liposomal dispersion for infusion.

Indications
Caelyx®
- Metastatic breast cancer (in patients with ↑ risk of cardiac toxicity).
- Advanced ovarian cancer after failure of platinum-based therapy.
- Progressive multiple myeloma.
- AIDS-related Kaposi's sarcoma.

Myocet®
- First-line metastatic breast cancer, in combination with cyclophosphamide.

Contraindications and precautions
- Monitor for myelosuppression.
- Fertility:
  - Advise barrier contraception during and for 3 months after therapy.
  - Risk of sterility—advise sperm storage for men.

☺ Undesirable effects
Common
- Alopecia (with Myocet®)
- Anorexia
- Constipation
- Diarrhoea
- Fatigue
- Mucositis
- Myelosuppression (grade 3 or 4 in 10–20%)
- Nausea
- Neutropenic fever
- PPE (45% with Caelyx®)
- Stomatitis
- Transaminitis
- Vomiting.

Uncommon
- Jaundice
- Pleural effusion
- Sepsis.

Drug interactions
Pharmacokinetic
- Caelyx® and Myocet® are not known to interact significantly with other medications. However, they are likely to interact with substances known to interact with conventional doxorubicin.

Pharmacodynamic
- When used with other myelosuppressive agents the risk of myelosuppression is ↑.

Dose

- Caelyx®: 50mg/m^2 once every 4 weeks (breast, ovarian cancer); 30mg/m^2 on day 4 of each 3-week cycle (myeloma, given with bortezomib).
- Myocet®: 60–75mg/m^2 once every 3 weeks, in combination with cyclophosphamide.

Dose adjustments

- Ovarian cancer: Caelyx® monotherapy is generally initiated at a dose of 40mg/m^2 (reduced rates of PPE and myelosuppression). In combination with carboplatin, Caelyx® dose is 30mg/m^2.

Additional information

There are no clinical trials of the use of Myocet® in patients with ovarian cancer.

Pharmacology

The active substance in Myocet® and Caelyx® is doxorubicin hydrochloride (HCL). The pegylated liposomes permit prolonged circulation of these agents in the bloodstream, and their small size (average diameter of 100nm) allows extravasation through defective tumour vasculature. At equivalent doses, the plasma concentration and AUC values of Caelyx®, which represent mostly pegylated liposomal doxorubicin HCL are significantly higher than those achieved with standard doxorubicin HCL.

Lomustine

CeeNU®/CCNU® (POM)

- Capsules: 10mg, 40mg, 100mg.

Indications

Usually used in combination regimens to treat the following:

- Primary or metastatic brain tumours (the 'C' in the PCV regimen)
- Small cell lung cancer
- Hodgkin disease
- Metastatic malignant melanoma.

Contraindications and precautions

- Severe renal impairment.
- Coeliac disease or wheat allergy.
- Can cause delayed myelosuppression lasting 6 weeks or more.
- Risk of pulmonary fibrosis. Patients should undergo baseline pulmonary function tests, along with frequent monitoring during treatment.
- Alcohol should be avoided whilst on lomustine chemotherapy.
- Fertility:
  - Advise barrier contraception during and for 3 months after therapy.
  - Risk of sterility—advise sperm storage for men.

☹ Undesirable effects

Common

- Delayed myelosuppression
- Fatigue
- Liver dysfunction
- Nausea/vomiting/anorexia.

Uncommon

- Diarrhoea
- Febrile neutropenia
- Transaminitis.

Rare

- Alopecia
- Cholestatic jaundice
- Interstitial pneumonia/pulmonary fibrosis
- Mild neurological symptoms (in combination with other antineoplastic drugs or radiotherapy)
- Renal toxicity
- Secondary malignancy
- Visual disturbance.

Drug interactions

Pharmacokinetic

- Concurrent treatment with phenobarbital can lead to ↑ metabolism and therefore reduced efficacy, via induction of microsomal liver enzymes.

Pharmacodynamic
- Concurrent treatment with other myelosuppressive agents, theophylline, or cimetidine increases the risk of myelosuppression.

Dose
- As monotherapy 120–130mg/m^2 PO every 6–8 weeks (either as a single dose or divided over 3 days).

Dose adjustments
- Reduce dose if patient develops leucopenia below 3.0×10^9/L or thrombocytopenia below 75×10^9/L.
- Give at a reduced dose when combined with other myelosuppressive drugs.

Additional information
- Patients should wear gloves when handling lomustine capsules.
- Swallow capsules whole with a large glass of water.
- Overdose should be treated immediately by gastric lavage.

Pharmacology
Lomustine is an alkylating nitrosourea. It is readily absorbed from the intestinal tract, with C_{max} reached 3 hours after oral administration. Lomustine is highly lipid soluble and therefore able to penetrate the blood–brain barrier. Lomustine is rapidly metabolized, with the serum half-life of the metabolites ranging from 16 hours to 2 days. The majority of metabolites are excreted via the kidneys within 24 hours.

Medroxyprogesterone

Provera® (POM)
- Tablet (scored): 2.5mg (30); 5mg (10); 10mg (10; 90); 100mg (60; 100); 200mg (30); 400mg (30).

Climanor® (POM)
- Tablet: 5mg (28).

Indications
- Endometrial carcinoma
- Renal cell carcinoma
- Carcinoma of breast in postmenopausal women
- ¥ Anorexia and cachexia[1]
- ¥ Sweating (associated with castration in men and women).[2,3]

Contraindications and precautions
- Medroxyprogesterone is contraindicated in patients with:
  - acute porphyria
  - angina
  - atrial fibrillation
  - cerebral infarction
  - DVT
  - endocarditis
  - heart failure
  - hypercalcaemia associated with bone metastases
  - impaired liver function or active liver disease
  - PE
  - thromboembolic ischaemic attack
  - thrombophlebitis
  - undiagnosed vaginal bleeding.
- May cause hypercalcaemia in patients with breast cancer and bone metastases.
- Unexpected vaginal bleeding during treatment should be investigated.
- Treatment with medroxyprogesterone can cause Cushingoid symptoms.
- Discontinue treatment if the following develop:
  - jaundice or deterioration in liver function
  - significant increase in blood pressure
  - new onset of migraine-type headache
  - sudden change in vision.
- Use with caution in patients with:
  - continuous treatment with relatively large doses continuously (monitor for signs hypertension, sodium retention, oedema)
  - depression
  - diabetes
  - epilepsy
  - hyperlipidaemia
  - hypertension
  - migraine
  - renal impairment.

- Patients may experience dizziness or drowsiness with medroxyprogesterone and should not drive (or operate machinery) if affected.

Adverse effects

The frequency is not defined, but reported adverse effects include:

- CHF
- Depression
- Dizziness
- Drowsiness
- Headache
- Hypercalcaemia
- Hypertension
- ↑ appetite
- Insomnia
- Malaise
- Menstrual irregularities
- Nervousness
- Oedema
- Reduced libido
- Thromboembolic disorders (e.g. PE, retinal thrombosis)
- Weight gain.

Drug interactions

Pharmacokinetic

- Medroxyprogesterone is a substrate of CYP3A4. Despite this, the clearance of medroxyprogesterone is believed to be approximately equal to hepatic blood flow. Therefore, medroxyprogesterone would not be expected to be affected by drugs that alter hepatic enzyme activity.
- Nonetheless, co-administration with drugs that are metabolized by, or affect the activity (induction or inhibition) of this pathway may lead to clinically relevant drug interactions and the prescriber should be aware that dosage adjustments may be necessary, particularly of drugs with a narrow therapeutic index.
- Avoid excessive amounts of grapefruit juice as it may increase the bioavailability of medroxyprogesterone through inhibition of intestinal CYP3A4.

Pharmacodynamic

- NSAIDs: ↑ risk of fluid retention.
- Warfarin: possible effect on bleeding times; INR should be monitored.

⚬⃗ Dose

Endometrial and renal cell carcinoma

- 200–600mg PO daily.

Breast carcinoma

- 400–1500mg PO daily.

¥ Anorexia and cachexia

- Initial dose 400mg PO every morning. Increase as necessary to a maximum of 1000mg PO daily (e.g. 500mg PO BD).

¥ Sweating

- 20mg PO OD for at least 4 weeks, then reduce to lowest possible dose that continues to relieve symptoms.

⚙ Dose adjustments

Elderly
- No dose adjustments are necessary.

Hepatic/renal impairment
- Although specific guidance is unavailable, the lowest effective dose should be used. Medroxyprogesterone is contraindicated in severe impaired liver function.
- Although specific guidance is unavailable, the lowest effective dose should be used. Medroxyprogesterone should be used with caution in patients with renal impairment.

Additional information
- As with corticosteroids and megestrol, the increase in body mass is likely to be due to retention of fluid or increase in body fat.
- Medroxyprogesterone has a catabolic effect on skeletal muscle which could further weaken the patient.

⊙ Pharmacology
- Medroxyprogesterone is a synthetic progestin and has the same physiologic effects as natural progesterone. It has a similar effect as megestrol.

References

1. Madeddu C, Macciò A, Panzone F, et al. Medroxyprogesterone acetate in the management of cancer cachexia. *Expert Opin Pharmacother* 2009; **10**(8): 1359–66.
2. Irani J, Salomon L, Oba R, et al. Efficacy of venlafaxine, medroxyprogesterone acetate, and cyproterone acetate for the treatment of vasomotor hot flushes in men taking gonadotropin-releasing hormone analogues for prostate cancer: a double-blind, randomized trial. *Lancet Oncol* 2010; **11**(2): 147–54.
3. Prior JC, Nielsen JD, Hitchcock CL, et al. Medroxyprogesterone and conjugated oestrogen are equivalent for hot flushes: A 1-year randomized double-blind trial following premenopausal ovariectomy. *Clin Sci* 2007; **112**(10): 517–25.

Megestrol

Megace® (POM)
- Tablet (scored): 160mg (30).

Generic (POM)
- Oral suspension: 40mg/5ml (150ml).

Indications
- Breast cancer
- ¥ Anorexia and cachexia[1]
- ¥ Sweating (associated with castration in men and women).[2]

Contraindications and precautions
- Use with caution in patients with:
  - history of thrombophlebitis
  - severe impaired liver function.
- Glucose intolerance and Cushing's syndrome have been reported with the use of megestrol. The possibility of adrenal suppression should be considered in all patients taking or withdrawing from chronic megestrol treatment. Glucocorticoid replacement treatment may be necessary.
- 2 case reports have associated its use in patients with prostate cancer with worsening disease.

Adverse effects
- The frequency is not defined, but commonly reported adverse effects include:
  - breakthrough uterine bleeding
  - headache
  - ↑ appetite and food intake
  - oedema
  - nausea
  - vomiting
  - weight gain.
- Other reported adverse effects include:
  - alopecia
  - carpal tunnel syndrome
  - Cushingoid facies
  - dyspnoea
  - heart failure
  - hot flushes
  - hyperglycaemia
  - hypertension
  - mood changes
  - PE
  - thrombophlebitis
  - tumour flare (with or without hypercalcaemia).

Drug interactions
Pharmacokinetic
- None stated.

Pharmacodynamic
• None stated.

♔ Dose
Breast cancer
• 160mg PO OD.

Endometrial cancer
• 40–320mg PO daily, in 2 or more divided doses.

¥ Anorexia and cachexia
• Initial dose 160mg PO OD, ↑ as necessary up to 800mg daily in 2 or more divided doses. Treatment should be continued for at least 6 weeks.

¥ Sweating
• 20–40mg PO every morning for at least 4 weeks.

♔ Dose adjustments
Elderly
• No dose adjustment is necessary.

Hepatic/renal impairment
• Undergoes complete hepatic metabolism. Although specific guidance is unavailable, the lowest effective dose should be used. Megestrol is contraindicated in severe impaired liver function.
• Doses adjustments are not necessary in renal impairment.

Additional information
• Although an oral suspension is available as a special order (e.g. Martindale Pharma—01277 266600), tablets can be crushed and dispersed in water immediately prior to administration.
• As with corticosteroids and medroxyprogesterone, the increase in body mass is likely to be due to retention of fluid or increase in body fat.
• Megestrol has a catabolic effect on skeletal muscle which could further weaken the patient.

⊙ Pharmacology
Megestrol is a synthetic progestin and has the same physiological effects as natural progesterone. It interferes with the oestrogen cycle and it suppresses LH release from the pituitary. It has a slight but significant glucocorticoid effect and a very slight mineralocorticoid effect. The precise mechanism of the effect on anorexic and cachexia is unknown. Megestrol has direct cytotoxic effects on breast cancer cells in tissue culture and may also have a direct effect on the endometrium.

References
1. Berenstein G, Ortiz Z. Megestrol acetate for treatment of anorexia-cachexia syndrome. *Cochrane Database Syst Rev* 2005; **2**: CD004310
2. Quella SK, Loprinzi CL, Sloan JA, *et al*. Long term use of megestrol acetate by cancer survivors for the treatment of hot flashes. *Cancer* 1998; **82**(9): 1784–8.

Melphalan

Alkeran® (POM)

- 2mg tablets, for oral use.
- 50mg, powder for reconstitution, for IV use.

Indications

- Conventional IV dose: multiple myeloma and ovarian cancer.
- Oral (may be used in combination with steroids and/or other chemotherapy agents): multiple myeloma and ovarian cancer.
- High IV dose (with or without haematopoietic stem cell transplant): multiple myeloma and childhood neuroblastoma.
- As regional intra-arterial perfusion: localized melanoma of the extremities and localized soft tissue sarcoma of the extremities.

Contraindications and precautions

- Patients with significant renal impairment.
- For patients receiving high-dose melphalan, assessment of co-morbidities and performance status should be carefully made.
- Fertility:
  - Advise barrier contraception during and for 3 months after therapy.
  - Risk of sterility—advise sperm storage for men.

☺ Undesirable effects

Common
- Diarrhoea
- Hair loss
- Mucositis (at high doses)
- Myelosuppression
- Nausea
- Reduced fertility in both men and women
- Vomiting.

Uncommon
- Rash.

Rare
- Interstitial pneumonitis and pulmonary fibrosis
- Secondary leukaemia.

Drug interactions

Pharmacokinetic
- Melphalan does not interact with many other drugs.

Pharmacodynamic
- Myelosuppressive effect potentiated by other myelosuppressive drugs.
- Associated mucositis may interfere with absorption of concurrently used oral medications.

⚕ Dose
- Regimen specific.
- High-dose IV is 200mg/m^2 (when used as single agent) or 140mg/m^2, e.g. when used as part of the BEAM regimen.
- Oral dose in combination with prednisolone: 7mg/m^2 daily for 4 days per cycle.

⚕ Dose adjustments
- Doses should be reduced in the setting of raised creatinine. Typically the dose is reduced by 50% if CrCl is <50ml/min and usually omitted if <30ml/min.

⟔ Pharmacology
Melphalan is a bifunctional alkylator causing DNA cross-links and inhibition of DNA replication.

Mercaptopurine

Puri-Nethol® (POM)
- 50mg tablets, containing 50mg of 6-mercaptopurine.

Indications
- Acute leukaemia
- Chronic granulocytic leukaemia.

Contraindications and precautions
- Hypersensitivity to any of the components.
- Fertility:
  - Advise barrier contraception during and for 3 months after therapy.
  - Risk of sterility—advise sperm storage for men.

☺ Undesirable effects
Common
- Biliary stasis/hepatotoxicity
- Fatigue
- Myelosuppression (leucopenia/thrombocytopenia more common than anaemia)
- Nausea and vomiting.

Uncommon
- Anaemia
- Febrile neutropenia
- Transaminitis.

Rare
- Alopecia (usually only thinning)
- Drug fever
- Hepatic necrosis
- Hypersensitivity reactions
- Skin rash.

Drug interactions
Pharmacokinetic
- Allopurinol: if administered concomitantly give only a quarter dose of mercaptopurine. Allopurinol decreases catabolism of mercaptopurine.
- Aminosalicylate derivatives: agents such as olsalazine and mesalazine inhibit the thiopurine methyltransferase (TPMT) enzyme and should therefore be used with caution.

Pharmacodynamic
- When used with other myelosuppressive agents the risk of myelosuppression is ↑.

⚕ Dose
- For adults and children usual starting dose is 2.5mg/kg per day, or 50–75mg/m^2 body surface area per day.

♣ Dose adjustments

- Consider reducing the dose in patients with hepatic or renal impairment.

Additional information

- There are individuals with an inherited deficiency of the enzyme TPMT, who may be unusually sensitive to the myelosuppressive effects of mercaptopurine. TPMT deficiency testing does not identify all patients at risk of severe toxicity; therefore blood counts should be carefully monitored.

♦ Pharmacology

Mercaptopurine is a sulphydryl analogue of the purine base hypoxanthine and acts as a cytotoxic antimetabolite. It is an inactive prodrug that requires cellular uptake and intracellular anabolism to thioguanine nucleotides for cytotoxicity. These cytotoxic metabolites inhibit *de novo* purine synthesis and purine nucleotide interconversions. Thioguanine nucleotides are also incorporated into nucleic acids, which contributes to the cytotoxic effects of the drug.

Mesna

Sodium-2-mercaptoethanesulphonate, Mesnex® (POM)

• Multidose vial for injection: 1000mg/10ml.

Indications

• Prevention of oxazaphosphorine (ifosfamide and cyclophosphamide)-induced haemorrhagic cystitis.

Contraindications

• History of hypersensitivity to mesna.

Precautions

• No evidence of teratogenicity.

☺ Undesirable effects

Virtually non-toxic at doses used for uroprotection.

Uncommon
• Abdominal pain
• Diarrhoea
• False positive urinary ketone analysis
• Nausea/vomiting
• Rash.

⚬ Dose

• Mesna should be given during and after oxazaphosphorine therapy until acrolein metabolites fall to non-toxic levels (usually 8–12 hours)

As uroprotectant for bolus oxazaphosphorine regimens
• Standard risk:
  • Mesna at 20% of ifosfamide dose immediately before, at 4 and 8 hours after ifosfamide.
  • Total mesna dose 60% (w/w) of total ifosfamide dose.
• High risk (previous oxazaphosphorine therapy/pelvic radiotherapy):
  • ↑ mesna dose to 40% of the oxazaphosphorine dose and give 4 doses at 3-hourly intervals (total mesna dose 160% (w/w) of oxazaphosphorine dose).
• Oral mesna regimens:
  • IV mesna bolus at 20% (w/w) ifosfamide dose immediately pre-ifosfamide *or* oral mesna at 40% (w/w) 2 hours prior to ifosfamide followed by oral mesna at 40% (w/w) total ifosfamide dose at 2 and 6 hours following ifosfamide.

As uroprotectant for infusional ifosfamide regimens
• IV bolus mesna at 20% (w/w) ifosfamide dose at start of infusion then infused mesna (100% w/w) concomitantly with infused ifosfamide. A further 12-hour infusion of mesna at 60% of the total dose of ifosfamide should be given after completion of ifosfamide infusion.
• Oral mesna is not recommended.

Drug interactions

• Antineoplastic effect of oxazaphosphorine/other antineoplastics is unaffected by mesna.

⚡ Dose adjustments

• None required.

⟜ Pharmacology

Following IV administration, mesna is rapidly oxidized to mesna-disulphide (dimesna), which remains in the intravascular compartment and is transported to the kidneys. Dimesna is reduced to the free thiol in renal tubuli, and reacts with the urotoxic acrolein metabolite of oxazaphosphorine to produce a nontoxic thioether. Elimination is almost exclusively renal and begins immediately following administration; excretion of both mesna and dimesna is generally complete within 8 hours. Oral administration of mesna is associated with urinary concentrations approximately half those following IV dosing, delay in urinary excretion of up to 2 hours and relative prolongation of excretion.

Methotrexate

Methotrexate (POM)
- Tablets: 2.5 and 10mg strengths.
- Injections: 5mg/2ml; 25mg/ml; 100mg/ml.

Indications
- Solid tumours, e.g. breast, lung, head and neck, bladder, cervical, ovarian and testicular cancer
- Soft tissue and osteogenic sarcomas
- Trophoblastic disease
- Acute leukaemias
- Lymphoma
- Severe uncontrolled psoriasis.

Contraindications and precautions
- Hypersensitivity to any of the components.
- Significant renal or hepatic impairment.
- Caution with concomitant use of other antifolate agents or drugs that reduce tubular secretion of methotrexate.
- Fertility:
  - Advise barrier contraception during and for 3 months after therapy.
  - Risk of sterility—advise sperm storage for men.

☺ Undesirable effects
Common
- Diarrhoea
- Myelosuppression (leucopenia/thrombocytopenia more common than anaemia)
- Nausea
- Ulcerative stomatitis.

Uncommon
- Acute or chronic interstitial pneumonitis
- Hepatic toxicity.

Rare
- Hypersensitivity reactions
- Pulmonary fibrosis
- Stevens–Johnson syndrome.

Drug interactions
Pharmacokinetic
- Methotrexate is extensively protein bound and can be displaced by drugs such as salicylates, hypoglycaemics, diuretics, sulphonamides, tetracyclines, p-aminobenzoic acid, giving the potential for ↑ toxicity.

Pharmacodynamic
- When used with other myelosuppressive agents the risk of myelosuppression is ↑.

♪ Dose

Methotrexate is active orally and parenterally. Dose is dependent on the indication, e.g.:

- Breast cancer: in combination with cyclophosphamide and 5-FU, IV methotrexate 40mg/m^2 on day 1 and 8.
- Choriocarcinoma: oral or IM 15–30mg for 5 days with rest periods of 1 or more weeks.
- Leukaemia: maintenance dosage of 20–30mg/m^2 orally or IM twice weekly.
- Osteosarcoma: starting dose 12g/m^2; high-dose treatment requires leucovorin rescue.

♪ Dose adjustments

- Dosing should be interrupted for neutropenia $<1.5 \times 10^9$/L or thrombocytopenia $<100 \times 10^9$/L. However, retreatment is guided by the indication and treatment intent.
- Dose reductions of 20% should be considered in significant renal or hepatic impairment.

Additional information

- Pleural effusions and ascites should be drained prior to initiation of methotrexate therapy, due to the risk of drug accumulation.

♦ Pharmacology

Methotrexate is an antimetabolite, which competitively inhibits the enzyme DHFR, resulting in impaired DNA synthesis and cellular replication. Actively proliferating tumour cells are thus more susceptible to the effects of this agent.

Mitomycin

Mitomycin-C Kyowa® (POM)

- Mitomycin 2mg, 10mg, 20mg, 40mg powder for solution for injection.

Indications

Mitomycin is recommended for certain types of cancer in combination with other drugs or after primary therapy has failed.

- As a single agent in the treatment of superficial bladder cancer.
- As a single agent and in combination with other drugs in metastatic breast cancer.
- In combination with other agents in advanced squamous cell carcinoma of the uterine cervix.
- As part of combination therapy in carcinoma of the stomach, pancreas, and lung (particularly non-small cell).
- As a single agent and in combination in liver cancer when given by the intra-arterial route.
- In combination with other cytotoxic drugs in the third-line treatment of metastatic colorectal cancer.
- As a single agent or part of combination therapy in cancer of the head and neck.
- Some activity as a single agent in cancer of the prostate.
- Possible roles in skin cancer, leukaemia, sarcomas.
- Used in combination with radiotherapy in, e.g. anal cancer.

Contraindications and precautions

Contraindications

- Previous hypersensitive or idiosyncratic reaction to mitomycin.
- Thrombocytopenia, coagulation, or bleeding disorders.

Cautions

- Hepatic or renal dysfunction: as adverse reactions may be enhanced.
- Bone marrow depression and bleeding tendency: as these may be exacerbated.
- Infections: as these may be aggravated due to bone marrow depression.
- Varicella: as fatal systemic disorders may occur.
- Administered with care when it is co-administered with other antineoplastic agents or irradiation. The adverse reactions of each drug may be enhanced, e.g. bone marrow depression.
- With vinca alkaloids: adverse reactions of shortness of breath and bronchospasm may be enhanced

☹ Undesirable effects

Common

- Leukopenia, thrombocytopenia, anaemia, bleeding tendency
- Malaise
- Nausea and vomiting, weight loss.

Uncommon

- Mouth ulcers
- Skin reactions, alopecia.

Rare
- Anaphylactoid reaction
- Myelodysplastic syndrome, AML, acute leukaemia
- Pulmonary oedema, interstitial pneumonia, and pulmonary fibrosis.

In addition to these effects, mitomycin can produce administration-related toxicity into the bladder, hepatic artery, and IV respectively:
- Cystitis, atrophy of the bladder, contracted bladder and calcinosis
- Liver and biliary tract disorders such as cholecystitis, cholangitis
- Pain, phlebitis, thrombus, induration/necrosis at the injection site.

Drug interactions
Pharmacokinetic
- No pharmacokinetic interactions have been described.

Pharmacodynamic
- When administered with other antineoplastic agents or irradiation, the adverse reactions may be enhanced, e.g. bone marrow depression.
- With vinca alkaloids shortness of breath/bronchospasm may be enhanced.
- Vaccines, live virus, should be used with extreme caution because normal defence mechanisms may be suppressed by mitomycin therapy.

,❁ Dose
- Usual dose 6–12mg/m^2 depending on route (higher for hepatic arterial route than IV) and frequency (4–6-weekly).
- A course ranging from 40–80mg is often required for a satisfactory response when used alone or in combination.
- In the treatment of superficial bladder tumours the usual dose is 20–40mg dissolved in 20–40ml of diluent, instilled into the bladder through a urethral catheter, weekly or 3 times a week for a total of 20 doses.

,❁ Dose adjustments
- Doses greater than 20mg/m^2 have not been shown to be more effective and are more toxic than lower doses and should not be used.

Additional information
- Local ulceration and cellulitis may be caused by tissue extravasation during IV injection and utmost care should be taken in administration. If extravasation occurs, follow local protocols.
- Intra-arterial administration may cause skin disorders such as pain, redness, erythema, blisters, erosion, and ulceration which may lead to skin/muscle necrosis.

⊕ Pharmacology
Mitomycin is an antitumour antibiotic that is activated in the tissues to an alkylating agent which disrupts DNA in cancer cells by forming a complex with DNA and also acts by inhibiting division of cancer cells by interfering with the biosynthesis of DNA.

Mitotane

Lysodren® (POM)
- Mitotane, white 500mg tablets.

Indications
- Symptomatic treatment of advanced (unresectable, metastatic or relapsed) adrenal cortical carcinoma.

Contraindications and precautions
Contraindications
- Patients with severe renal or hepatic impairment.

Cautions
Caution should be exercised in patients who have the following pre-exististent problems:
- Hepatic impairment: carefully monitor in patients with mild to moderate liver dysfunction.
- Renal impairment: carefully monitor in patients with mild to moderate renal dysfunction.
- Elderly populations: there is no experience on the use of mitotane in elderly patients, so data are insufficient to give a dose recommendation in this group.
- Large metastatic masses should be surgically removed as far as possible before starting mitotane treatment, in order to minimize the risk of infarction and haemorrhage in the tumour due to a rapid shrinkage.
- Mitotane should be temporarily discontinued immediately following shock, severe trauma, or infection, since adrenal suppression is its prime action.

☺ Undesirable effects
Common
- ↑ cholesterol/triglycerides
- Confusion, paraesthesia, vertigo, sleepiness, ataxia
- Diarrhoea, nausea, vomiting, mucositis, abdominal pain, stomatitis
- Fatigue
- ↑ hepatic enzymes ALT/AST
- Rash.

Uncommon
- Autoimmune hepatitis
- Mental impairment, movement disorder, dizziness, headache
- Thrombocytopenia, anaemia.

Rare
- Hyperpyrexia
- Maculopathy, retinal toxicity, lens opacity, visual impairment.

Drug interactions
Pharmacokinetic
- Mitotane must not be given in combination with spironolactone since the latter may block the action of mitotane, although why is not clear.

- Mitotane has been reported to accelerate the metabolism of warfarin through hepatic microsomal enzyme induction, leading to an increase in dose requirements for warfarin. Therefore monitor closely.
- Has an inductive effect on cytochrome P450 enzymes. Therefore, the plasma concentrations of the substances metabolized via cytochrome P450 may be modified.

Pharmacodynamic
- Mitotane can cause CNS undesirable effects at high concentrations and this should be borne in mind when co-prescribing medicinal products with CNS depressant action.

☕ Dose
- Start with 2–3g mitotane per day and ↑ progressively (e.g. at 2-week intervals) until mitotane plasma levels reach the therapeutic window 14–20mg/L. Dose adjustment is aimed to reach this therapeutic window which ensures optimal effect of mitotane with acceptable safety.

☕ Dose adjustments
- Dose adjustments should be made according to plasma levels and endeavouring to keep these within the therapeutic window.

Additional information
- Fat-rich food: data with various mitotane formulations suggest that administration with fat-rich food enhances absorption of mitotane.
- Hormone binding protein: mitotane has been shown to increase plasma levels of hormone binding proteins (e.g. sex hormone-binding globulin and corticosteroid-binding globulin). This should be taken into account when interpreting the results of hormonal assays and may result in gynaecomastia.
- Before the initiation of the treatment: large metastatic masses should be surgically removed as far as possible before starting mitotane treatment, in order to minimize the risk of infarction and haemorrhage in the tumour due to a rapid cytotoxic effect of mitotane.

✈ Pharmacology
Mitotane is an adrenal cytotoxic active substance, although it can apparently also cause adrenal inhibition without cellular destruction. Its biochemical mechanism of action is unknown. Available data suggest that mitotane modifies the peripheral metabolism of steroids and that it also directly suppresses the adrenal cortex. The administration of mitotane alters the extra-adrenal metabolism of cortisol in humans, leading to a reduction in measurable 17-hydroxy corticosteroids, even though plasma levels of corticosteroids do not fall. Mitotane apparently causes ↑ formation of 6-beta-hydroxy cholesterol.

After IV administration, 25% of the dose is excreted as metabolites within 24 hours. Following discontinuation of mitotane treatment, it is slowly released from storage sites in fat, leading to reported terminal plasma half-lives ranging from 18 to 159 days.

Mitoxantrone

Mitoxantrone hydrochloride, Novantrone® (POM)

- Vials for injection: 20mg/10ml.

Indications

- Castration-resistant advanced/metastatic prostate cancer
- Metastatic breast cancer
- Non-Hodgkin lymphoma
- Adult acute non-lymphocytic leukaemia.

Contraindications

- History of hypersensitivity to mitoxantrone
- Significant bone marrow suppression is a relative contraindication.

Precautions

- Cardiac monitoring with interval echocardiography recommended if:
    - history of left ventricular dysfunction
    - previous anthracycline treatment
    - previous radiotherapy encompassing the heart
    - cumulative mitoxantrone dose >160mg/m^2.
- ❶ Vesicant: extravasation may result in tissue necrosis.
- Fertility:
    - Advise barrier contraception during and for 3 months after therapy.
    - Risk of sterility—advise sperm storage for men.

☺ Undesirable effects

Common

- Alopecia
- ↑ bilirubin
- Mucositis
- Myelosuppression (nadir 10–14 days)—dose-limiting toxicity
- Nausea and vomiting (low emetic risk)

Uncommon

- Cardiac failure (↑ in patients with risk factors or high cumulative dose—📖 Precautions, see above)
- Cough with or without dyspnoea
- Diarrhoea, abdominal pain
- ↑ hepatic transaminases
- Rash.

Rare

- Blue discoloration of sclerae
- Seizures.

Drug interactions

- Cardiotoxic drugs: avoid if possible.

♣ Dose

Castration-resistant prostate cancer
- 12mg/m^2 every 3–4 weeks in combination with prednisolone 5mg BD.

Metastatic breast cancer/non-Hodgkin lymphoma
- 12–14mg/m^2 every 3–4 weeks (↓ dose in pretreated patients or diminished performance status).

♣ Dose adjustments

Combination therapy
- Dose reduction by 2–4mg/m^2 is recommended when used in combination therapy.

Hepatic impairment
- Bilirubin >60micromol/L with good performance status: give 60% dose.
- Bilirubin >60micromol/L with poor performance status: omit.

Myelosuppression
- Dose reduction by 2mg/m^2 is recommended if nadir WBC <1.5 × 10^6/mm^3 or nadir platelets <50 × 10^6/mm^3.

⊙ Pharmacology

Mitoxantrone is an antitumour antibiotic with structural similarity to anthracyclines, which is believed to exert its antiproliferative effect by DNA intercalation. Mitoxantrone is rapidly distributed to tissues following IV administration, with 80% bound to plasma proteins. Mitoxantrone undergoes hepatic metabolism and is excreted unchanged in bile (30%) and urine (10%). Drug elimination is slow with a mean half-life of 12 days.

Oxaliplatin

Eloxatin® (POM)

- Concentrate for solution for infusion. Clear, colourless solution, free from visible particles; a pH in the range of 3.5–6.5 and 125–175mOsm/L osmolarity.

Indications

Oxaliplatin in combination with 5-FU and folinic acid is indicated for:

- Adjuvant treatment of stage III (Dukes' C) colon cancer after complete resection of primary tumour.
- Treatment of metastatic colorectal cancer.

  Also now commonly replaces cisplatin in the treatment of gastric cancer.

Contraindications and precautions

- Oxaliplatin is contraindicated in patients who:
  - have a known history of hypersensitivity to oxaliplatin or to its excipient
  - are breastfeeding
  - have myelosuppression prior to starting first course, as evidenced by baseline neutrophils $<2 \times 10^9$/L and/or platelet count of $<100 \times 10^9$/L
  - have a peripheral sensitive neuropathy with functional impairment prior to first course
  - have a severely impaired renal function (CrCl <30ml/min).

Caution

- Patients with a history of allergic reaction to platinum compounds should be monitored for allergic symptoms. In case of an anaphylactic-like reaction to oxaliplatin, the infusion should be immediately discontinued and appropriate symptomatic treatment initiated. Oxaliplatin rechallenge is contraindicated.

☺ Undesirable effects

Common

- Anaemia, neutropenia, thrombocytopenia, lymphopenia
- Fatigue, injection site pain
- Hepatic enzyme increase
- Nausea, vomiting, abdominal pain
- Peripheral sensory neuropathy, headache.

Uncommon

- Dizziness
- Febrile neutropenia
- Rash
- Thromboembolism
- Visual disturbance.

Rare

- Haemolytic anaemia
- Immunoallergic thrombocytopenia

- Interstitial lung disease
- Reversible visual field and acuity loss
- RPLS.

Drug interactions

Pharmacokinetic
- None described.

Pharmacodynamic
- A synergistic cytotoxic action has been observed in combination with 5-FU both *in vitro* and *in vivo*.

♣ Dose

- The dose of oxaliplatin is 85mg/m^2 intravenously by infusion over 2 hours every 2 weeks, or 130mg/m^2 every 3 weeks. Oxaliplatin is always given in combination with 5-FU or capecitabine because of the proven synergy.

♣ Dose adjustments

If neurological symptoms (paraesthesia, dysaesthesia) occur, the following recommended oxaliplatin dosage adjustment should be based on the duration and severity of these symptoms:
- If symptoms last >7 days and are troublesome, the subsequent oxaliplatin dose should be reduced from 85mg/m^2 to 65mg/m^2 (metastatic setting) or 75mg/m^2 (adjuvant setting).
- If paraesthesia without functional impairment persists until the next cycle, the subsequent oxaliplatin dose should be reduced from 85mg/m^2 to 65mg/m^2 (metastatic setting) or 75mg/m^2 (adjuvant setting).
- If paraesthesia with functional impairment persists until the next cycle, oxaliplatin should be discontinued.
- If grade 4 diarrhoea, grade 3–4 neutropenia (neutrophils <1.0 × 10^9/L), grade 3–4 thrombocytopenia (platelets <50 × 10^9/L) occur, the dose of oxaliplatin should be reduced from 85mg/m^2 to 65mg/m^2 (metastatic setting) or 75mg/m^2 (adjuvant setting), in addition to any 5-FU dose reductions required.

☼ Pharmacology

Oxaliplatin belongs to a new class of platinum-based compounds in which the platinum atom is complexed with 1,2-diaminocyclohexane ('DACH') and an oxalate group. It is a single enantiomer, (*SP*-4–2)-[(1R,2R)-cyclohexane-1,2-diamine-k*N*, k*N′*] [ethanedioato(2-)-k*O*^{1}, k*O*^{2}] platinum. Studies on the mechanism of action show that the aqua-derivatives resulting from the biotransformation of oxaliplatin, interact with DNA to form both inter- and intrastrand cross-links, resulting in the disruption of DNA synthesis leading to cytotoxic and antitumour effects.

Paclitaxel

Paclitaxel (POM)
- 6mg/ml concentrate for solution for infusion.

Abraxane® (POM)
- 5mg/ml powder for suspension for infusion.

Indications
- Adjuvant treatment of ovarian cancer (in combination with carboplatin).
- Advanced ovarian cancer.
- Adjuvant treatment of breast cancer.
- Locally advanced or metastatic breast cancer (the only indication for Abraxane®).
- Advanced NSCLC.
- ¥ Metastatic melanoma.

Contraindications and precautions
- Patients must be pretreated with corticosteroids, antihistamines, and H2 antagonists.
- Fertility:
  - Advise barrier contraception during and for 3 months after therapy.
  - Risk of sterility—advise sperm storage for men.

☺ Undesirable effects
Common
- Alopecia
- Arthralgia and myalgia
- Diarrhoea
- Fatigue
- Infection
- Mild skin and nail changes
- Minor hypersensitivity reactions
- Myelosuppression (grade 3 or 4 in 10–20%)
- Nausea
- Peripheral neuropathy
- Transaminitis
- Vomiting.

Uncommon
- Significant hypersensitivity reactions
- Febrile neutropenia.

Rare
- Pseudomembranous colitis
- Cardiac conduction abnormalities
- Febrile neutropenia.

Drug interactions
Pharmacokinetic
- Caution should be exercised when administering paclitaxel with other CYP3A4 or CYP2C8 inhibitors, such as erythromycin, fluoxetine, or inducers such as rifampicin, carbamazepine.

Pharmacodynamic
- When used with other myelosuppressive agents the risk of myelosuppression is ↑.

₄ᴊ Dose
- Recommended IV dosage: paclitaxel 175mg/m² every 3 weeks.
- ¥ Weekly paclitaxel: 80mg/m² weekly until disease progression; for 3 weeks out of 4, or weekly for 6 weeks out of 8.
- Abraxane® 260mg/m² administered intravenously every 3 weeks.

₄ᴊ Dose adjustments
- Patients with severe hepatic dysfunction should not be treated with paclitaxel.
- Patients experiencing severe neutropenia or severe peripheral neuropathy should receive a dose reduction of 20% for subsequent doses.

Additional information
- ¥ There is increasing use of weekly paclitaxel schedules for the treatment of ovarian and breast cancers. Metronomic paclitaxel has additional antiangiogenic effects; however, haematological and neurological toxicity is more pronounced.
- Abraxane® is an albumin-bound nanoparticle formulation of paclitaxel with enhanced tumour permeability. It is currently licensed for the treatment of metastatic breast cancer.

⊕ Pharmacology
Paclitaxel is an antimicrotubule agent that promotes microtubular stability and prevents depolymerization, blocking cells in the G2/M phase of the cell cycle. There is also evidence that weekly administration of paclitaxel has an antiangiogenic mode of action.

Panitumumab

Vectibix® (POM)

- Panitumumab 20mg/ml concentrate for solution for infusion.

Indications

Panitumumab (Vectibix®) is indicated for the treatment of patients with wild-type KRAS metastatic colorectal cancer (mCRC):

- In first-line in combination with 5-FU and oxaliplatin.
- In second-line in combination with 5-FU and irinotecan.
- As monotherapy after failure of fluoropyrimidine-, oxaliplatin-, and irinotecan-containing chemotherapy regimens.

Contraindications and precautions

Contraindications

- History of severe/life-threatening hypersensitivity reactions to the drug.
- Interstitial pneumonitis or pulmonary fibrosis.

Cautions

- Patients on a controlled sodium diet as the drug contains 0.150mmol sodium per ml of concentrate.
- Panitumumab should not be administered in combination with bevacizumab-containing chemotherapy regimens.
- Patients with a history of keratitis, ulcerative keratitis, or severe dry eye as can exacerbate these conditions
- ECOG 2 performance status as a positive benefit–risk balance has not been documented in patients with ECOG 2 performance status.
- Patients with hepatic or renal impairment—no data available.

☺ Undesirable effects

Common

- Fatigue
- GI: diarrhoea, nausea, vomiting, abdominal pain, anorexia, stomatitis
- Hypomagnesaemia
- Skin reactions: rash, dermatitis acneiform, pruritus, erythema, dry skin, paronychia.

Uncommon

- Infusion reaction
- Keratitis.

Rare

- Anaphylactic reaction
- Ulcerative keratitis.

Drug interactions

Pharmacokinetic

- The pharmacokinetics of irinotecan and its active metabolite, SN-38, are not altered when the panitumumab is co-administered.; nor vice versa.

Pharmacodynamic
- Panitumumab should not be administered in combination with IFL (irinotecan, folinic acid, 5-FU) chemotherapy or with bevacizumab-containing chemotherapy. A high incidence of severe diarrhoea was observed when panitumumab was administered in combination with the IFL regimen and ↑ toxicity and deaths were seen when panitumumab was combined with bevacizumab and chemotherapy.

Dose
- Always as an IV infusion.
- 6mg/kg of bodyweight given once every 2 weeks. Prior to infusion, panitumumab should be diluted in 0.9% sodium chloride injection to a final concentration not to exceed 10mg/ml.

Dose adjustments
- For skin symptoms grade 3 or grade 4:
  - 1st occurrence, hold 1 or 2 doses and if improved continue at same dose but if no improvement, discontinue.
  - 2nd occurrence, hold 1 or 2 doses and if improved reduce dose to 80%, but if no improvement, discontinue.
  - 3rd occurrence, hold 1 or 2 doses and if improved reduce dose to 60% and if no improvement, discontinue.
  - 4th occurrence, discontinue.
- In the event of acute onset or worsening pulmonary symptoms, panitumumab treatment should be interrupted and a prompt investigation of these symptoms should occur. If interstitial lung disease is diagnosed, panitumumab should be permanently discontinued and the patient should be treated appropriately.
- If a severe or life-threatening reaction occurs during an infusion or at any time post infusion (e.g. presence of bronchospasm, angio-oedema, hypotension, need for parenteral medication, or anaphylaxis), panitumumab should be permanently discontinued.
- If a diagnosis of ulcerative keratitis is confirmed, treatment with panitumumab should be interrupted or discontinued. If keratitis is diagnosed, the benefits/risks of continuing treatment should be carefully considered.

Additional information
Human IgG is known to cross the placental barrier, and panitumumab may therefore be transmitted from the mother to the developing fetus. In women of childbearing potential, appropriate contraceptive measures must be used.

Pharmacology
Panitumumab is a recombinant, fully human IgG2 monoclonal antibody that binds with high affinity and specificity to human EGFR. EGFR is a transmembrane glycoprotein that is a member of a subfamily of type I receptor tyrosine kinases including EGFR (HER1/c-ErbB-1), HER2, HER3, and HER4). Panitumumab binds to the ligand binding domain of EGFR and inhibits receptor autophosphorylation induced by all known EGFR ligands. Binding of panitumumab to EGFR results in internalization of the receptor, inhibition of cell growth, induction of apoptosis, and ↓ interleukin 8 and VEGF production.

Pazopanib

Votrient® (POM)

- Film-coated tablets: 200mg, 400mg.

Indications

- First-line therapy of metastatic renal cancer
- STS.

Contraindications

- Hypersensitivity to pazopanib.

Precautions

- Risk of hepatic failure: check LFTs before therapy and monitor monthly during treatment.
- Hypertension: discontinue therapy if persistent ↑ blood pressure >140/90mmHg despite antihypertensive medication.
- Use with caution in patients with cardiac dysfunction.
- Risk of QT prolongation: use with caution in patients treated with drugs that prolong QT interval.
- Risk of delayed wound healing due to VEGF inhibition: recommend discontinuation 7 days before surgery and restart when healing satisfactory.
- Risk of teratogenicity: advise barrier contraception during and for 3 months after therapy.

☹ Undesirable effects

Common

- Abdominal pain and diarrhoea
- Anorexia
- Change in hair colour
- Fatigue
- Hepatic transaminitis
- Hypertension
- Hypothyroidism
- Myelosuppression
- Nausea and vomiting
- Rash.

Uncommon

- Cardiac dysfunction
- Hepatic failure (📖 Precautions, see above for monitoring)
- Hypophosphataemia, hypomagnesaemia
- QT prolongation.

Rare

- GI perforation.

Drug interactions

- Cytochrome P450 inhibitors: ↑ pazopanib concentrations.
- Simvastatin: concurrent use ↑ incidence of transaminitis (ALT 3 × ULN 27% vs. 14%).

- PPIs/H2-receptor antagonists: ↑ gastric pH associated with ↓ pazopanib bioavailability.

Dose
- 800mg OD.

Dose adjustments
Elderly
- Limited data on patients >65 years. Though no difference in metabolism noted, manufacturer recommends clinical decision.

Renal impairment
- No alteration in dose recommended if GFR >30ml/min, advise caution if GFR <30ml/min as limited data.

Hepatic impairment
- Mild hepatic impairment (normal bilirubin, any ALT level or bilirubin up to 1.5× ULN regardless of the ALT value): recommended starting dose 800mg OD.
- Moderate hepatic impairment (defined as an elevation of bilirubin >1.5 to 3× ULN regardless of the ALT values): recommended dose 200mg OD.

Pharmacology
Pazopanib is a tyrosine kinase inhibitor that targets VEGFR-1, -2, and -3, platelet-derived growth factor receptor (PDGFR)- α and - β, and stem cell factor (c-KIT). By blocking ligand-induced receptor phosphorylation, pazopanib blocks mitogenic and antiapoptotic signalling and inhibits tumour and blood vessel growth. Pazopanib is well absorbed orally with maximum plasma concentrations obtained at a median of 3.5 hours following administration, with >99% circulating drug bound to plasma proteins. Metabolism is primarily by CYP3A4 and elimination via faeces with mean half-life of 30.9 hours. <4% pazopanib is eliminated renally.

Pemetrexed

Alimta® (POM)
- Powder for solution for infusion: 100mg, 500mg.

Indications
- Mesothelioma (in combination with cisplatin).
- Advanced/metastatic NSCLC of non-squamous histology:
  - In combination with cisplatin as first-line therapy.
  - As maintenance monotherapy following non-progression of disease on platinum-based first-line chemotherapy.

Contraindications
- History of hypersensitivity to pemetrexed
- Renal impairment (GFR < 45ml/min)
- Breastfeeding.

Precautions
Concomitant vitamins
- Pretreatment with folic acid and vitamin B12 is required to reduce toxicities:
  - At least 5 doses of folic acid (350–1000mcg PO daily) should be taken in the 7 days preceding the 1st dose of pemetrexed and should continue until 21 days after the final pemetrexed dose.
  - IM vitamin B12 (1000mcg) should be given in the week prior to pemetrexed and subsequently should be given every 3 cycles.

Renal impairment
- Patients with mild to moderate renal insufficiency (GFR 45–79ml/min) should avoid taking NSAIDs and aspirin (>1.3g daily) for 2 days before, during and subsequent to pemetrexed therapy.
- Fertility:
  - Advise barrier contraception during and for 3 months after therapy.
  - Risk of sterility—advise sperm storage for men.

☺ Undesirable effects
Common
- Anorexia
- Diarrhoea
- Fatigue
- Febrile neutropenia
- ↑ hepatic transaminases
- Myelosuppression
- Nausea and vomiting (low emetic risk)
- Rash.

Uncommon
- Cardiovascular/cerebrovascular events
- Peripheral ischaemia
- Renal failure.

Rare
- Colitis
- Interstitial pneumonitis.

Drug interactions
- Nephrotoxic agents: (see 📖 Precautions, p.186).
- Pemetrexed pharmacokinetics are not altered by concomitant administration of cisplatin.
- Cytochrome P450 inhibitors/inducers: no significant interaction predicted.

💊 Dose
In combination with cisplatin
- 500mg/m^2 followed by 75mg/m^2 cisplatin on day 1 of a 21-day cycle.

As monotherapy
- 500mg/m^2 on day 1 of a 21-day cycle.

💊 Dose adjustments
Based on myelosuppression during previous cycle
- Nadir absolute neutrophil count (ANC) <0.5 × 10^3 cells/mm^3 and nadir platelets >50 × 10^3 cells/mm^3: 75% previous dose.
- Nadir platelets <50 × 10^3 cells/mm^3 irrespective of ANC: 75% previous dose.
- Nadir platelets >50 × 10^3 cells/mm^3 with bleeding, irrespective of ANC: 50% previous dose.

Non-haematological toxicity
- G3/4 non-mucositis: 75% previous dose.
- G3/4 mucositis: 50% previous dose.

Investigations prior to therapy
- Pemetrexed should only be given providing the following parameters are met:
  - >1.5 × 10^3 cells/mm^3
  - Platelets >100 × 10^3 cells/mm^3
  - Bilirubin <1.5 × ULN
  - Alkaline phosphatase/ALT/AST <3 × ULN (unless due to liver metastases in which case <5 × ULN).

⊙ Pharmacology
Pemetrexed is a multitargeted antifolate that targets cell replication through inhibition of TS, DHFR, and glycinamide ribonucleotide formyl-transferase (GARFT)—folate-dependent enzymes critical for *de novo* nucleotide biosynthesis. ~80% of injected pemetrexed is bound to plasma proteins, with 70–90% of drug excreted unchanged in the urine within 24 hours of administration.

Pentostatin

Nipent® (POM)
- 10mg powder for solution for injection: IV injection.

Indications
- Hairy cell leukaemia (as a single agent).

Contraindications and precautions
- Highly immunosuppressive (myelosuppressive and lymphotoxic) so ensure no active infection prior to treatment.
- Contraindicated in renal impairment (CrCl <60ml/min).

☺ Undesirable effects
Common
- Anaemia
- Fatigue
- Febrile neutropenia
- Fever
- Leucopenia
- Nausea
- Thrombocytopenia.

Uncommon
- Asthma
- Diarrhoea
- Rash
- Renal impairment
- Stomatitis
- Tumour lysis syndrome.

Rare
- Transfusion-associated graft-versus-host disease.

Drug interactions
Pharmacokinetic
- Pentostatin does not interact widely with other drugs.

Pharmacodynamic
- Myelosuppressive effect potentiated by other myelosuppressive drugs.
- Not recommended to be used with fludarabine due to ↑ incidence of fatal pulmonary complications.

Dose
- 4mg/m^2 IV every 14 days.

Dose adjustments
- Contraindicated in moderate to severe renal failure (CrCl <60ml/min).
- Little information on use in patients with liver disease. Contraindicated in moderate to severe liver disease.

Additional information

Patients should receive irradiated blood products for life after receiving pentostatin to avoid the risk of transfusion-associated graft-versus-host disease.

◈ Pharmacology

Pentostatin is a potent transition state inhibitor of adenosine deaminase (ADA). It also leads to direct inhibition of RNA synthesis and DNA damage, all of which contribute to cytotoxicity. ADA is most active in lymphocytes, explaining selective killing of lymphoid cells.

Plicamycin

Mithramycin, Mithracin® (POM)

- Powder for solution for infusion: 2.5g.

Indications

- Testicular seminoma and NSGCT
- Hypercalcaemia of malignancy.

Contraindications

- History of hypersensitivity to plicamycin.
- Concomitant varicella or herpes zoster infection (may result in severe, potentially fatal, generalized disease).

Precautions

- Facial flushing, epistaxis, and prolongation of PT predict ↑ risk of fatal bleeding—treatment should be withheld if present.
- ❶ Vesicant: extravasation may be result in significant tissue necrosis.
- Fertility:
  - Advise barrier contraception during and for 3 months after therapy.
  - Risk of sterility—advise sperm storage for men.

☺ Undesirable effects

Common

- Bleeding episodes (12% overall, risk of fatal bleeding in up to 6% patients receiving >30mcg/kg/24 hours)
- Nausea and vomiting
- Thrombocytopenia (nadir 5–10 days).

Uncommon

- Headache, dizziness
- ↑ hepatic transaminases
- Proteinuria, ↑ serum creatinine
- Rash
- ↑ serum bilirubin
- ↓ serum Ca^{2+}.

Drug interactions

- Concomitant calcitonin administration: may result in significant hypocalcaemia.

♣ Dose

Testicular cancer

- 25–30mcg/kg/24 hours for 8–10 days.

Hypercalcaemia of malignancy

- 25–30mcg/kg/24 hours given 1–3 times a week.

♣ Dose adjustments

Bleeding risks

- Consider alternate day dosing if signs predicting bleeding are present to reduce risk.

Hepatic impairment
• If used for hypercalcaemia of malignancy reduce dose to 12mcg/kg.

Renal impairment
• Reduce dose if GFR <60ml/min.

Oedema
• Use ideal body weight for dosing.

⊙ Pharmacology

Plicamycin is an antitumour antibiotic poorly absorbed by mouth. Following IV administration, distribution is to the liver, kidney, bone, and cerebrospinal fluid (CSF). Metabolism is hepatic with an elimination half-life of ~2 hours. 25–40% of plicamycin is eliminated unchanged in the urine.

Procarbazine

Procarbazine (POM)
- 50mg tablets.

Indications
- Wide range of tumours as part of multidrug regimens, especially breast cancer and lung cancer.

Contraindications and precautions
- Cyclophosphamide is contraindicated in haemorrhagic cystitis.
- Use with caution on patients with hepatic or renal failure.
- Avoid dosing in patients with severe infections.
- Fertility:
  - Advise barrier contraception during and for 3 months after therapy.
  - Risk of sterility—advise sperm storage for men.

☺ Undesirable effects
Common
- Allergic skin reaction
- Alopecia
- Anorexia
- Fatigue
- Leucopenia
- Nausea
- Rash
- Thrombocytopenia
- Vomiting.

Uncommon
- Disordered liver function
- Infertility (which may be irreversible)
- Jaundice.

Rare
- Convulsions
- Hallucinations.

Drug interactions
Pharmacokinetic
- Weak MAO inhibition may potentiate the effects of narcotic analgesics, anticholinergic drugs, anaesthetics, and some antihypertensives.

Pharmacodynamic
- ↑ agranulocytosis has been reported when procarbazine is administered concurrently with clozapine.
- Use with enzyme-inducing antiepileptics is associated with an ↑ risk of hypersensitivity reactions to procarbazine.

⚗ Dose
- As monotherapy the procarbazine dose should be ↑ gradually to a maximum 300mg daily in evenly divided doses.

- As part of multidrug regimens procarbazine is usually given for the 1st 10–14 days of each 4- to 6-week cycle at 100mg/m^2 PO OD (rounded to the nearest 50mg).

♣ Dose adjustments
- Treatment should be interrupted for allergic skin reactions.
- Procarbazine dosing should be interrupted where platelets fall below 80 × 10^{12}/ml or white cells below 3 × 10^{12}/ml until recovery.

◈ Pharmacology
Procarbazine, a methylhydrazine derivative, is a cytostatic agent with weak MAO inhibitor properties. Its exact mode of action on tumour cells is unknown.

Raltitrexed

Tomudex® (POM)
- Powder for solution for injection: 2mg per vial.

Indications
- The palliative treatment of advanced colorectal cancer where 5-FU and folinic acid-based regimens are either not tolerated or inappropriate.

Contraindications and precautions
Contraindications
- Severe renal or severe hepatic impairment.

Cautions
Caution should be exercised in the following patient populations:
- Elderly patients are more vulnerable to the toxic effects of raltitrexed. Extreme care should be taken to ensure adequate monitoring of adverse reactions, especially signs of GI toxicity.
- A proportion of the raltitrexed is excreted via faecal route; caution in patients with mild to moderate hepatic impairment.
- ↑ incidence of grade 3 or 4 adverse reactions in patients with moderate renal impairment. For patients with abnormal serum creatinine, before the 1st or any subsequent treatment, a CrCl should be performed or calculated. For reduced CrCl the following adjustments should be made: Clearance of 55–65ml/min, administer 75% of the full dose every 4 weeks; clearance of 25–54ml/min, administer 50% of full dose every 4 weeks; clearance of <25ml/min, no treatment.

☺ Undesirable effects
Common
- Asthenia, fatigue
- Diarrhoea, nausea, vomiting, anorexia, stomatitis, dehydration, change in taste
- Flu-like symptoms
- Neutropenia, anaemia, thrombocytopenia
- Rash.

Uncommon
- Alopecia
- ↑ liver enzymes and bilirubin
- Infection.

Rare
- Desquamation.

Drug interactions
Pharmacokinetic
No specific clinical drug–drug interaction studies have been conducted in humans.

Pharmacodynamic
- Folinic acid and folic acid must not be given immediately prior to or during administration of raltitrexed as it may interfere with its action.

♣ Dose
- 3mg/m² given intravenously, as a single, short, IV infusion (in 50–250ml of either 0.9% sodium chloride solution or 5% glucose solution), over a 15min period. In the absence of toxicity, treatment may be repeated every 3 weeks.

♣ Dose adjustments
In the event of toxicity withhold until toxic effects regress. In particular, signs of GI toxicity (diarrhoea or mucositis) and haematological toxicity (neutropenia or thrombocytopenia) should have completely resolved before subsequent treatment is allowed.

Based on the worst grade of GI and haematological toxicity observed on the previous treatment and provided that such toxicity has completely resolved, the following dose reductions are recommended:
- Grade 3 haematological toxicity: 25% dose reduction; grade 4 haematological toxicity: 50% dose reduction.
- Grade 2 GI toxicity: 25% dose reduction; grade 3 GI toxicity: 50% dose reduction.
- Grade 4 GI toxicity (diarrhoea or mucositis) or in the event of a grade 3 GI toxicity associated with grade 4 haematological toxicity: treatment should be discontinued.

Additional information
- Patients with grade 4 GI toxicity (diarrhoea or mucositis) or grade 3 GI toxicity associated with grade 4 haematological toxicity require aggressive supportive management with IV hydration and bone marrow support.
- It is essential that the dose reduction scheme should be adhered to since the potential for life-threatening and fatal toxicity increases if the dose is not reduced or treatment not stopped as appropriate.

♦ Pharmacology
Raltitrexed is a folate analogue belonging to the family of antimetabolites and has potent inhibitory activity against the enzyme TS. It acts as a direct and specific TS inhibitor, a key enzyme in the synthesis of thymidine triphosphate (TTP), a nucleotide required exclusively for DNA synthesis. Inhibition of TS leads to DNA fragmentation and cell death. Raltitrexed is transported into cells via a reduced folate carrier and is then extensively polyglutamated by the enzyme folyl polyglutamate synthetase to polyglutamate forms that are retained in cells and are even more potent inhibitors of TS.

Regorafenib

Stivarga® (POM)

- 40mg light pink film coated tablets.

Indications

- Regorafenib is indicated for the treatment of patients with metastatic colorectal cancer who have been previously treated with fluoropyrimidine-, oxaliplatin-, and irinotecan-based chemotherapy, an anti-VEGF therapy, and, if KRAS wild type, an anti-EGFR therapy.

Contraindications and precautions

Contraindications

- None.

Cautions

- Stop regorafenib before surgery. Discontinue if there is wound dehiscence.
- Withhold regorafenib for new or acute cardiac ischaemia/infarction.
- Can cause fetal harm.
- Not recommended in severe hepatic failure nor tested in severe renal failure.

☺ Undesirable effects

Common

- ↓ appetite and food intake
- Asthenia/fatigue
- Diarrhoea
- Dysphonia
- Haemorrhage
- Hypertension
- Infection
- Mucositis
- PPE, rash
- Weight loss.

Uncommon

- Abnormal INR
- Alopecia
- Dry mouth
- Dry skin
- Gastro-oesophageal reflux
- Hyperuricaemia
- Hypocalcaemia
- Hypokalaemia
- Hypomagnesaemia
- Hyponatraemia
- Hypophosphataemia
- Leukopenia
- Musculoskeletal stiffness
- Proteinuria
- Taste disorder
- ↑ transaminases/lipase/ amylase/ hypothyroidism.

Rare

- GI perforation
- Hypertensive crisis
- Myocardial infarction
- Myocardial ischaemia
- RPLS
- Severe liver injury.

Drug interactions

Pharmacokinetic

- Strong CYP3A4 inducers ↓ the mean exposure of regorafenib, ↑ the mean exposure of the active metabolite M-5, and resulted in no

change in the mean exposure of the active metabolite M-2. Avoid concomitant use of strong CYP3A4 inducers.
- Co-administration of strong CYP3A4 inhibitors ↑ the mean exposure of regorafenib and ↓ the mean exposure of the active metabolites M-2 and M-5. Avoid concomitant use of strong inhibitors of CYP3A4 activity.

Dose
- The recommended dose is 160mg regorafenib (four 40mg tablets) taken orally once daily for the first 21 days of each 28-day cycle. Continue treatment until disease progression or unacceptable toxicity.

Dose adjustments

Interrupt regorafenib for the following:
- Grade 2 PPE that is recurrent or does not improve within 7 days despite dose reduction or interrupt for grade 3 PPE.
- Symptomatic grade 2 hypertension.
- Any grade 3 or 4 adverse reaction.

Reduce the dose of regorafenib to 120mg:
- For the first occurrence of grade 2 PPE of any duration.
- After recovery of any grade 3 or 4 adverse reaction.
- For grade 3 AST/ALT elevation.

Reduce the dose of regorafenib to 80mg:
- For re-occurrence of grade 2 PPE at the 120mg dose.
- After recovery of any grade 3/4 adverse reaction at the 120mg dose.

Discontinue regorafenib permanently for the following:
- Any occurrence of AST/ALT >20 × ULN.
- Any occurrence of AST/ALT >3 × ULN with concurrent bilirubin >2 × ULN.
- Re-occurrence of AST or ALT >5 × ULN despite dose reduction to 120mg.
- For any grade 4 adverse reaction.

Additional information
Severe drug-induced liver injury with fatal outcome occurred in 0.3% of regorafenib-treated patients across all clinical trials. Obtain liver function tests (ALT, AST and bilirubin) before initiation of regorafenib and monitor at least every 2 weeks during the first 2 months of treatment. Thereafter, monitor monthly or more frequently as clinically indicated.

Pharmacology
Regorafenib is a small-molecule inhibitor of multiple membrane-bound and intracellular kinases. In *in vitro* biochemical or cellular assays, regorafenib or its major human active metabolites M-2 and M-5 inhibited the activity of RET, VEGFR1, VEGFR2, VEGFR3, KIT, PDGFR- α, PDGFR- β, FGFR1, FGFR2, TIE2, DDR2, Trk2A, Eph2A, RAF-1, BRAF, BRAFV600E, SAPK2, PTK5, and Abl at concentrations of regorafenib that have been achieved clinically. Regorafenib is metabolized by CYP3A4 and UGT1A9.

Rituximab

MabThera® (in Europe, POM), Rituxan® (in the USA, POM)

- 100mg or 500mg vials: concentrate for IV infusion.

Indications

- Stage II–IV follicular lymphoma in combination with chemotherapy in previously untreated patients or in relapsed disease.
- Maintenance therapy for patients with stage II–IV follicular lymphoma responding to rituximab chemotherapy induction.
- CD20-positive, diffuse large B-cell lymphoma in combination with chemotherapy for first-line treatment.
- CLL in combination with chemotherapy in both previously untreated and relapsed patients.
- ¥ Frequently also used in CD20-positive non-follicular low-grade non-Hodgkin lymphoma (single agent or in combination with chemotherapy).
- ¥ Monotherapy, or in combination with chemotherapy, in post-transplant lymphoproliferative disorder.

Contraindications and precautions

- May cause reactivation of hepatitis B—check serology before treatment.

☺ Undesirable effects

Common
- Infusion reactions: fever, rigors, rash.

Uncommon
- Cytokine release syndrome characterized by bronchospasm, angio-oedema, fevers, chills, rigors.
- Delayed onset neutropenia.

Rare
- Progressive multifocal leucoencephalopathy.

Drug interactions

Pharmacokinetic
- No significant interactions.

Pharmacodynamic
- No significant interactions.

⚕ Dose

- $375mg/m^2$ is the standard dose in most indications although this is ↑ to $500mg/m^2$ in CLL.

✣ Pharmacology

Rituximab is a chimeric anti-CD20 monoclonal antibody. CD20 is widely expressed by B cells (but not terminally differentiated plasma cells). Binding initiates a number of events that can lead to apoptosis. Direct stimulation of apoptosis, recruitment of antibody-dependent cell cytotoxicity, and complement fixation are all involved.

Sorafenib

Nexavar® (POM, Bayer)

- 200mg film-coated tablets.

Indications

- Hepatocellular carcinoma
- Metastatic renal cell cancer.

Contraindications and precautions

- Antibiotics affecting gut microflora may reduce the bioavailability of sorafenib.
- Use with caution in patients who have, or may develop prolongation of QTc, such as patients with a congenital long QT syndrome, those treated with a high cumulative dose of anthracycline therapy, patients taking medicinal products that lead to QT prolongation, and those with electrolyte disturbances.

☺ Undesirable effects

Very common

- Alopecia
- ↑ amylase or lipase
- Diarrhoea
- Erythema
- Fatigue
- Haemorrhage
- Hypertension (including, rarely, crisis)
- Hypophosphataemia
- Itching
- Lymphopenia
- Nausea
- PPE
- Rash
- Vomiting.

Common

- Flu like illness
- Anorexia
- Arthralgia
- Cardiac failure
- Constipation
- Cytopenia
- Depression
- Dermatitis/dry skin
- Erectile dysfunction
- Fever
- Hypocalcaemia
- Myalgia
- Myocardial ischaemia/infarction
- Sensory neuropathy
- Tinnitus.

Uncommon

- Cholecystitis
- Dehydration
- Eczema
- Folliculitis
- Gastritis
- Gynaecomastia
- Hypersensitivity reactions
- Hyponatraemia
- Interstitial lung disease
- Jaundice
- Pancreatitis
- RPLS
- Squamoproliferative skin lesions
- Thyroid dysfunction (hypo- and hyper-).

Rare side effects include:
- Anaphylaxis
- Angio-oedema
- Drug-induced hepatitis
- QT prolongation
- Rhabdomyolysis
- Stevens–Johnson syndrome
- Toxic epidermal necrolysis.

Drug interactions

Pharmacokinetic
- Sorafenib inhibits glucuronidation via UGT1A1 and UGT1A9.
- Co-administration of neomycin interferes with enterohepatic recycling of sorafenib, reducing bioavailability. Other antibiotics affecting microorganisms with glucuronidase activity may have a similar effect.

⚖ Dose
- 400mg PO BD, taken without food.

⚖ Dose adjustments
- Dosing should be interrupted for persistent toxicities, and resumed at full dose or with a decrease to 400mg once a day once these have resolved to grade 1 or better.

⊕ Pharmacology
Sorafenib is a multikinase inhibitor that decreases tumour cell proliferation *in vitro*. Sorafenib inhibits tumour growth of a broad range of human tumour xenografts accompanied by a reduction in tumour angiogenesis. Sorafenib inhibits the activity of targets in tumour cells (CRAF, BRAF, V600E BRAF, c-KIT, and FLT-3) and in the tumour vasculature (CRAF, VEGFR-2, VEGFR-3, and PDGFR-β).

Streptozocin

Zanosar® (POM)
- Streptozocin. Pale yellow powder for solution for injection.

Indications
- Treatment of metastatic islet cell carcinoma of the pancreas: responses have been obtained with both functional and non-functional carcinomas. Because of its inherent renal toxicity, therapy with this drug should be limited to patients with symptomatic or progressive metastatic disease.

Contraindications and precautions
Cautions
- Caution should be exercised in patients with pre-existing renal disease: use requires a judgement by the physician of potential benefit as opposed to the known risk of serious renal damage.

☺ Undesirable effects
Common
- Asthenia
- Fatigue
- GI: diarrhoea, nausea, vomiting, anorexia, dehydration
- Injection site reaction
- Liver: elevated AST/ALT
- Renal: azotaemia, anuria, hypophosphatemia, glycosuria, and renal tubular acidosis (📖 Dose, see below).

Uncommon
- Haematological: anaemia
- Neurological: confusion, depression.

Rare
- Haematological: neutropenic sepsis, severe thrombocytopenia
- Metabolic: hypoglycaemic coma.

Drug interactions
Pharmacokinetic
- Streptozocin has been reported to prolong the elimination half-life of doxorubicin and may lead to severe bone marrow suppression.

Pharmacodynamic
- Streptozocin may demonstrate additive toxicity when used in combination with other cytotoxic drugs.

⚗ Dose
Daily schedule
The recommended dose for daily IV administration is 500mg/m^2 of body surface area for 5 consecutive days every 6 weeks until maximum benefit or until treatment-limiting toxicity is observed. Dose escalation on this schedule is not recommended.

Weekly schedule

The recommended initial dose for weekly IV administration is 1000mg/m^2 of body surface area at weekly intervals for the first 2 courses (weeks). In subsequent courses, drug doses may be escalated in patients who have not achieved a therapeutic response and who have not experienced significant toxicity with the previous course of treatment. However, *a single dose of 1500mg/m^2 body surface area should not be exceeded* as a greater dose may cause azotaemia. When administered on this schedule, the median time to onset of response is about 17 days and the median time to maximum response is about 35 days. The median total dose to onset of response is about 2000mg/m^2 body surface area and the median total dose to maximum response is about 4000mg/m^2 body surface area.

Dose adjustments
• No specific dose adjustments for toxicity are described.

Additional information
Renal toxicity is dose related and cumulative and may be severe or fatal. Other major toxicities are nausea and vomiting which may be severe and at times treatment-limiting. In addition, liver dysfunction, diarrhoea, and haematological changes have been observed in some patients. Streptozocin is mutagenic in animal models and therefore the cost: benefit ratio for an individual patient must be carefully assessed.

Pharmacology
Streptozocin inhibits DNA synthesis in bacterial and mammalian cells. In bacterial cells, a specific interaction with cytosine moieties leads to degradation of DNA. The biochemical mechanism leading to mammalian cell death has not been definitely established; streptozocin inhibits cell proliferation at a considerably lower level than that needed to inhibit precursor incorporation into DNA or to inhibit several of the enzymes involved in DNA synthesis. Although streptozocin inhibits the progression of cells into mitosis, no specific phase of the cell cycle is particularly sensitive to its lethal effects.

Sunitinib

Sunitinib
- Hard gelatin capsules: 12.5mg, 25mg, 37.5mg, and 50mg.

Indications
- Metastatic renal cell cancer
- Unresectable and/or metastatic GIST
- Unresectable and/or metastatic well-differentiated pancreatic neuroendocrine tumours.

Contraindications and precautions
- Co-administration with potent CYP3A4 inducers should be avoided as it may decrease plasma concentration of sunitinib.
- Co-administration with potent CYP3A4 inhibitors should be avoided as it may increase plasma concentration of sunitinib.
- Hypersensitivity to the active substance or any of the excipients is a contraindication.

☺ Undesirable effects
Common
- Anaemia
- Diarrhoea
- Dry skin
- Fatigue/asthenia
- Hypertension
- Hypothyroidism
- Nausea/vomiting
- Neutropenia
- Poor appetite
- PPE
- Skin discoloration
- Taste disturbance
- Thrombocytopenia.

Uncommon
- Cardiac disorders
- Epistaxis
- Hepatic dysfunction
- Intestinal perforation
- Pancreatitis
- Respiratory failure.

Rare
- Hepatitis/hepatic failure
- ONJ
- Thromboembolic events
- QT prolongation.

Drug interactions
Pharmacokinetic
- Sunitinib is metabolized by CYP3A4, and is affected by co-administration of other drugs that are inhibitors or inducers of CYP3A4.

Pharmacodynamic
- Sunitinib is not licensed in combination with other chemotherapeutic drugs.

⚖ Dose
- For GIST and metastatic renal cell cancer, the dose is 50mg PO OD, for 4 consecutive weeks, followed by a 2-week rest period (Schedule 4/2) to comprise a complete cycle of 6 weeks.

- For pancreatic neuroendocrine tumours, the recommended dose is 37.5mg PO OD continuously.

Dose adjustments

- For GIST and metastatic renal cell cancer, dose adjustments in 12.5mg steps according to tolerability and recurrence of toxicities. The dose should not exceed 75mg or go below 25mg.
- For pancreatic neuroendocrine tumours, dose adjustments in 12.5mg steps.

Additional information

- Sunitinib may be taken with or without food.

Pharmacology

Sunitinib inhibits multiple receptor tyrosine kinases implicated in tumour growth, new blood vessel formation, and metastatic progression of cancer. Sunitinib is metabolized by cytochrome P450 CYP3A4 to an active metabolite SU12662 which is further metabolized by CYP3A4 to an inactive compound.

Tamoxifen

Generic (POM)
- Tablet: 10mg (30); 20mg (30).
- Oral solution: 10mg/5ml (150ml).

Indications
- Breast cancer
- Anovulatory infertility.

Contraindications and precautions
- Tamoxifen is linked to an ↑ risk of endometrial changes including hyperplasia, polyps, cancer, and uterine sarcoma. Any patient with unexpected or abnormal gynaecological symptoms, especially vaginal bleeding, should be investigated.
- There is a 2–3× increase in risk of VTE in patients taking tamoxifen. Long-term anticoagulant prophylaxis may be necessary for some patients who have multiple risk factors for VTE
- ↑ bone pain, tumour pain, and local disease flare are sometimes associated with a good tumour response shortly after starting tamoxifen, and generally subside rapidly.
- Avoid combination with CYP2D6 inhibitors because these may interact with tamoxifen resulting in a poorer clinical outcome.

Adverse effects
The frequency is not defined, but reported adverse effects include:

- Alopecia
- Fluid retention
- Headache
- Hot flushes
- Hypercalcaemia (may occur on initiation of therapy)
- Light-headedness
- Liver enzyme changes
- Mood changes (e.g. depression)
- Nausea
- Pruritus vulvae
- Tumour flare (e.g. bone pain)
- Vaginal bleeding
- Vaginal discharge.

Drug interactions
Pharmacokinetic
- Tamoxifen is a major substrate of CYP2C8/9, CYP2D6, and CYP3A4. Co-administration with drugs that are metabolized by, or affect the activity (induction or inhibition) of these pathways, may lead to clinically relevant drug interactions and the prescriber should be aware that dosage adjustments may be necessary, particularly of drugs with a narrow therapeutic index.
- Co-administration with certain CYP2D6 inhibitors (e.g. paroxetine) has been shown to reduce the plasma levels of the potent antioestrogen endoxifen. The precise clinical significance of this interaction is presently unknown, but the UK Medicines and Healthcare products Regulatory Agency has recently advised co-administration of CYP2D6 inhibitors should be avoided. Patients who are CYP2D6 PMs may possibly have poorer than expected outcomes with tamoxifen.

Pharmacodynamic
- Warfarin: ↑ anticoagulant sensitivity. Mechanism unknown.

⚡ Dose
Breast cancer
- 20mg PO OD. No evidence exists for superiority of higher doses.

⚡ Dose adjustments
Elderly
- Usual adult doses can be used.

Hepatic/renal impairment
- No specific guidance is available for use in liver impairment. In view of the extensive metabolism of tamoxifen, the patient may be more susceptible to adverse effects and/or treatment failure.
- No dose adjustments are necessary for patients with renal impairment.

⊙ Pharmacology
- Tamoxifen is a non-steroidal antioestrogen that has both oestrogen antagonist and agonist activity. It acts as an antagonist on breast tissue and as an agonist in the endometrium, bone, and lipids. The precise mechanism of action is unknown, but the effect of tamoxifen is mediated by its metabolites, 4-hydroxytamoxifen and endoxifen. The formation of these active metabolites is catalysed by CYP2D6. It is also metabolized by several other cytochrome P450 isoenzymes (CYP2C8/9 and CYP3A4).

Temozolomide

Temodar® (POM)
- Capsules: 5mg, 20mg, 100mg, 140mg, 180mg, 250mg.

Indications
- Malignant glioma at recurrence or on progression after standard therapy.
- First-line treatment of malignant glioma concomitant with radiotherapy and subsequently as monotherapy.
- ¥ Melanoma.

Contraindications and precautions
- Temozolomide should not be used in patients with myelosuppression.
- Patients should be given prophylactic antiemetics.
- Fertility:
  - Advise barrier contraception during and for 3 months after therapy.
  - Risk of sterility—advise sperm storage for men.

☺ Undesirable effects
Common
- Alopecia (usually only thinning)
- Constipation
- Fatigue
- Headache
- Myelosuppression (grade 3 or 4 in 10–20%)
- Nausea/vomiting/anorexia
- Rash.

Uncommon
- Diarrhoea
- Dyspnoea/cough
- Febrile neutropenia
- Transaminitis.

Rare
- Hypersensitivity reactions
- Opportunistic infection (with longer durations of treatment)
- Stevens–Johnson syndrome
- Toxic epidermal necrolysis.

Drug interactions
Pharmacokinetic
- Temozolomide does not interact significantly with other medications.

Pharmacodynamic
- When used with other myelosuppressive agents the risk of myelosuppression is ↑.

♣ Dose

- With radiotherapy: 75mg/m^2/day PO OD for 42 days.
- As monotherapy: 150–200mg/m^2/day PO OD for 5 consecutive days every 4 weeks.

♣ Dose adjustments

- When given with radiotherapy dosing should be interrupted for neutropenia <1.5 × 10^9/L or thrombocytopenia <100 × 10^9/L and discontinued where there is neutropenia <0.5 × 10^9/L or thrombocytopenia <10 × 10^9/L, or for grade 3 non-haematological toxicities.
- Retreatment as monotherapy is guided by the nadir blood counts taken on day 22 of each treatment cycle.

Additional information

- Capsules should be taken whilst fasting, and should be swallowed whole.

◈ Pharmacology

Temozolomide is rapidly absorbed from the upper GI tract. It is hydrolysed at physiological pH to form the active moiety MTIC and acts by methylating DNA. The most important DNA lesion for temozolomide's antitumour activity is considered to be at the O6 position on guanine, although N7 methylguanine may make a contribution. MTIC is excreted renally and has low protein binding.

Thalidomide

Thalidomide Celgene® (POM)

- Capsule: 50mg (28).

Indications

- Multiple myeloma
- ¥ Cancer cachexia[1]
- ¥ Paraneoplastic sweating[2]
- ¥ Management of tumour-related gastric bleeding.[3]

Contraindications and precautions

- Must not be used in the following circumstances:
  - Pregnant women
  - Women of childbearing potential unless all the conditions of the Thalidomide Celgene® Pregnancy Prevention Programme are met (see manufacturer's SPC).
- The conditions of the Thalidomide Celgene® Pregnancy Prevention Programme (see manufacturer's SPC) must be fulfilled for all male and female patients.
- For women of childbearing potential, prescriptions for thalidomide should not exceed 4 weeks. Dispensing should occur within 7 days of the date of issue. For other patients, supply should be limited to 12 weeks.
- Thromboembolism and peripheral neuropathy have been reported to occur with thalidomide. Use cautiously with drugs that may increase the risk of thromboembolism or peripheral neuropathy.

- Patients prescribed thalidomide are at an ↑ risk of arterial and VTE (including cerebrovascular events, DVT, myocardial infarction, and PE). Thromboprophylaxis should be administered for at least the first 5 months of treatment especially in patients with additional thrombotic risk factors (e.g. LMWH, warfarin).
- Thalidomide must be discontinued if the patient experiences a thromboembolic event. Once the patient is stabilized on appropriate anticoagulant treatment, thalidomide can be re-started.
- The anticoagulant must be continued throughout the course of thalidomide treatment.
- Peripheral neuropathy can present with the following symptoms:
  - Abnormal coordination
  - Dysaesthesia
  - Paraesthesia
  - Weakness.
- Patients presenting with these symptoms should be assessed according the manufacturer's SPC. Treatment may be withheld or discontinued.

- Unused capsules should be returned to a pharmacy.
- Thalidomide may modify reactions and patients should be advised not to drive (or operate machinery) if affected.

Adverse effects

Very common

- Anaemia
- Constipation
- Dizziness
- Drowsiness
- Dysaesthesia
- Leucopenia
- Lymphopenia

- Neutropenia
- Paraesthesia
- Peripheral neuropathy
- Peripheral oedema
- Thrombocytopenia
- Tremor.

Common

- Bradycardia
- Cardiac failure
- Confusion
- DVT
- Depression
- Dry mouth
- Dyspnoea

- Malaise
- Nausea/vomiting
- Pneumonia
- PE
- Pyrexia
- Toxic skin eruptions
- Weakness.

Drug interactions

Pharmacokinetic

- Thalidomide does not appear to be metabolized by the liver. Clinically significant pharmacokinetic drug interactions have not been reported.

Pharmacodynamic

- Antiarrhythmics: ↑ risk of bradycardia.
- Bisphosphonates: ↑ risk of renal impairment (in treatment of multiple myeloma).
- CNS depressants: risk of excessive sedation.
- Dexamethasone: may increase the risk of toxic skin reactions, immunosuppression, and thromboembolic events.
- Epoetins: ↑ risk of thromboembolic events.
- NSAIDs: theoretical ↑ risk of thromboembolic events.

⚕ Dose

Multiple myeloma

- 200mg PO every night for 6-week cycle.
- Patient can receive a maximum of 12 cycles.

¥ *Cancer cachexia*

- 50–100mg PO every night.
- Further dose increases up to 200mg PO every night may be considered.

¥ *Paraneoplastic sweating*

- 50–100mg PO every night.
- Further dose increases up to 200mg PO every night may be considered.

¥ *Management of tumour-related gastric bleeding*

- 100–300mg PO every night.
- Used in combination with other agents such as sucralfate and PPIs.

🔁 Dose adjustments

Elderly
- No dose adjustments are necessary.

Hepatic/renal impairment
- There are no specific instructions for dose adjustment in liver or renal impairment. The lowest effective dose should be prescribed and the patient should be closely monitored.

Additional information
- The capsule must not be broken/opened; it must be swallowed whole.

⊕ Pharmacology
Thalidomide is an immunomodulatory agent that also has anti-inflammatory and antiangiogenic properties. The mechanism of action of thalidomide is not completely understood, although it has been shown to inhibit the synthesis of tumour necrosis factor (TNF)-A and modulates the effects of other cytokines. The exact metabolic pathway of thalidomide is unknown, but it is believed not to involve the cytochrome P450 system, but undergoes non-enzymatic hydrolysis in plasma.

References

1. Davis M, Lasheen W, Walsh D, *et al.* A Phase II Dose Titration Study of Thalidomide for Cancer-Associated Anorexia. *J Pain Symptom Manage* 2012; **43**(1): 78–86.
2. Deaner PB. The use of thalidomide in the management of severe sweating in patients with advanced malignancy: trial report. *Palliat Med* 2000; **14**(5): 429–31.
3. Lambert K, Ward J. The use of thalidomide in the management of bleeding from a gastric cancer. *Palliat Med* 2009; **23**(5): 473–5.

Thiotepa

Tepadina® (POM)
- 15mg or 100mg powder for concentration for solution for infusion.

Indications
- As conditioning treatment, in combination with other chemotherapy drugs and with or without total body irradiation, prior to allogeneic or autologous haematopoietic progenitor cell transplantation (HPCT) in haematological malignancies.
- As high-dose chemotherapy, in combination with other chemotherapy drugs, and with HPCT support in the treatment of some solid tumours (breast, ovarian, germ cell, and CNS tumours).

Contraindications and precautions
- Use with caution in patients with hepatic or renal impairment and those with a history of cardiac disease. Liver, renal, and cardiac function should be monitored regularly whilst on treatment with thiotepa.
- Must be given after, not concurrently with, cyclophosphamide.
- Concomitant use with yellow fever vaccine is contraindicated due to risk of fatal generalized vaccine-induced disease. Use of other live attenuated vaccines is not recommended for the same reason.
- Contraindicated during pregnancy and breastfeeding.

☹ Undesirable effects
Common (>10%)
- Acute/chronic GVHD
- Alopecia
- Anorexia
- Anxiety
- Arthralgia
- Blurred vision
- Cardiac arrhythmias
- Colitis
- Confusion
- Conjunctivitis
- Convulsions
- Diarrhoea
- Dizziness
- Encephalopathy
- Epistaxis
- Haemorrhagic cystitis
- Headaches
- Hyperglycaemia
- Hypertension
- Liver dysfunction
- Lymphoedema
- Myalgia
- Myelosuppression
- Nausea
- Oesophagitis
- Ototoxicity
- Pruritus
- Pyrexia
- Rash
- Stomatitis
- Thromboembolic disease
- Vaginal bleeding.

In paediatric patients
- Endocrine dysfunction
- Growth retardation.

Uncommon (1–10%)
- Cataracts
- Extrapyramidal disorder
- Intracranial aneurysm
- Menopausal symptoms
- Pneumonitis
- Pulmonary oedema
- Reduced fertility.

Rare (<1%)

- Cardiomyopathy
- Erythrodermic psoriasis
- Gastric ulceration
- Hallucinations
- Toxic shock syndrome.

Drug interactions

Pharmacokinetic

- Concomitant use of inhibitors or inducers of CYP2B6 or CYP3A4, as well as substrates of CYP2B6 should be monitored closely.
- Can decrease levels/efficacy of phenytoin if administered concomitantly.

Pharmacodynamic

- Risk of fatal generalized vaccine-induced disease if used concomitantly with yellow fever vaccine.
- In patients previously treated with radiotherapy, 3 or more cycles of chemotherapy or prior progenitor cell transplant there may be an ↑ risk of developing hepatic veno-occlusive disease.
- ↑ risk of pulmonary toxicity in patients treated with similarly toxic chemotherapy, e.g. busulfan, fludarabine, cyclophosphamide.
- Previous brain irradiation or craniospinal irradiation may contribute to severe toxic reactions, such as encephalopathy.
- When used with other myelosuppressive agents, in particular ciclosporin or tacrolimus, the risk of myelosuppression is ↑.

♪ Dose

- Dosage varies according to combination, type of HPCT, type of disease, and use in adults or children.
- In haematological malignancies: generally 125–300mg/m^2/day
- In solid tumours: generally 120–250mg/m^2/day
- Usually administered for 2–5 days prior to HPCT.

♪ Dose adjustments

- No specific dose adjustments are recommended.
- No dose adjustment is recommended for elderly patients.

Additional information

- Administered intravenously as a 2–4-hour infusion via a central venous catheter.

♦ Pharmacology

Thiotepa is an alkylating agent, related chemically and pharmacologically to nitrogen mustard. Oral absorption is variable, so it is generally administered intravenously, although it can also be administered intravesically. Thiotepa crosses the blood–brain barrier, with CSF exposure nearly equivalent to that achieved in plasma. Thiotepa is rapidly and extensively metabolized by the liver, undergoing oxidative desulphuration via the cytochrome P450 CYP2B and CYP3A isoenzyme families. Elimination half-life varies from 1.5 to 4.1 hours. Metabolites are excreted via urine.

Topotecan

Hycamtin® (POM)

- Capsules: 0.25mg and 1mg hard capsules.
- Topotecan powder: 1mg and 4mg powder for concentrate for infusion.

Indications

- Topotecan IV monotherapy: metastatic carcinoma of the ovary after failure of first-line or subsequent therapy.
- Relapsed small cell lung cancer.
- Hycamtin® capsules monotherapy: relapsed small cell lung cancer when re-treatment with first-line regimen is not considered appropriate.
- Topotecan in combination with cisplatin: stage IVB cervical cancer and carcinoma of cervix recurrent after radiotherapy.

Contraindications and precautions

- Haematological toxicity is dose related and FBCs should be monitored regularly.
- Dosing recommendations for Hycamtin® capsules in patients with CrCl of <60ml/min have not been established.
- Fertility:
- Advise barrier contraception during and for 3 months after therapy.
- Risk of sterility—advise sperm storage for men.

☺ Undesirable effects

Common

- Alopecia
- Anorexia
- Constipation
- Diarrhoea
- Fatigue
- Febrile neutropenia
- Hypersensitivity and rash
- Infection
- Myelosuppression
- Nausea
- Pruritus
- Vomiting.

Uncommon

- Hyperbilirubinaemia
- Neutropenic colitis.

Rare

- Anaphylaxis
- Interstitial lung disease.

Drug interactions

Pharmacokinetic

- Ciclosporin (an inhibitor of ABCB1, ABCC1 [MRP-1], and CYP3A4) administered with oral topotecan increases topotecan exposure.

Pharmacodynamic

- When used with other myelosuppressive agents the risk of myelosuppression is ↑.

♣ Dose
- With cisplatin 50mg/m^2 on day 1: topotecan 0.75mg/m^2/day as a 30min infusion on days 1, 2, and 3, repeated every 3 weeks for 6 courses or until progression.
- As monotherapy: 1.5mg/m^2/day administered by IV infusion over 30min daily for 5 consecutive days every 3 weeks.
- Hycamtin® capsules: 2.3mg/m^2/day daily for 5 consecutive days every 3 weeks, until disease progression.

♣ Dose adjustments
- Topotecan (IV): dose reductions for severe neutropenia (neutropenia <0.5 × 10^9/L for 7 days), neutropenic fever/sepsis, or recurrent neutropenic delays are recommended, e.g. to 1.25mg/m^2/day and subsequently to 1.0mg/m^2/day.
- Topotecan (IV): moderate renal impairment—consider dose reductions. If CrCl 20–30ml/min, topotecan (IV) dose reduced to 0.75mg/m^2/day for 5 consecutive days.
- Topotecan (PO): dose reductions for severe neutropenia (neutropenia <0.5 × 10^9/L for 7 days), neutropenic fever/sepsis, or recurrent neutropenic delays are recommended, e.g. to 1.9mg/m^2/day.
- Topotecan (PO): patients with a CrCl of <60ml/min may be more susceptible to toxicity but there are no data on the safety of oral administration in this group.
- Topotecan (PO): reduce dose by 0.4mg/m^2/day for ≥grade 2 diarrhoea.

Additional information
- Capsules should be swallowed whole.

♦ Pharmacology
Topotecan is a semisynthetic derivative of camptothecin, a natural product extracted from tree bark. The antitumour activity of topotecan involves inhibition of topoisomerase-1, a nuclear enzyme intimately involved in DNA replication. Topotecan intercalates between DNA bases and disrupts DNA replication leading ultimately to cell death.

Toremifene

Fareston® (POM)

- Tablet 60mg.

Indications

- Treatment of hormone-dependent metastatic breast cancer in postmenopausal patients.

Contraindications

- △ Risk of QT prolongation, avoid in the following:
  - Congenital or acquired QT prolongation
  - Electrolyte disturbance
  - Clinically relevant bradycardia/heart failure with ↓ LVEF
  - Concurrent use of drugs that prolong QT interval.
- Pre-existing endometrial hyperplasia
- Severe liver failure
- Hypersensitivity to toremifene

Precautions

- ❶ Risk of QT prolongation (▢ Contraindications, see above).
- Gynaecological examination recommended before and each year while on therapy (risk of endometrial neoplasia).
- Use not recommended in patients with history of life-threatening thromboembolic disease.
- Close monitoring of patients with bone metastases is required when starting therapy due to risk of hypercalcaemia.

☺ Undesirable effects

Common
- Hot flushes
- Sweats
- Depression
- Nausea/vomiting
- Uterine bleeding, leucorrhoea.

Uncommon
- Endometrial hypertrophy
- Thromboembolism
- Constipation
- Weight gain.

Rare
- Endometrial hyperplasia/cancer
- ↑ hepatic transaminases
- Jaundice.

Drug interactions

- ❶ Agents prolonging QT interval.
- Drugs that reduce renal calcium excretion: ↑ risk of hypercalcaemia.
- Cytochrome P450 inducers: may ↑ toremifene metabolism resulting in ↓ serum levels. Doubling of daily dose may be required.

Dose
- 60mg daily.

Dose adjustments
Hepatic impairment
- Use with caution.

Renal impairment
- No dose adjustment required.

Pharmacology
Toremifene is a non-steroidal triphenylethylene derivative that competes with oestradiol for binding of oestrogen receptors and inhibits oestrogen-induced cellular proliferation. Following oral administration toremifene is rapidly absorbed and reaches peak serum concentrations within 3 to 4 hours. Toremifene is extensively bound to serum proteins (92% albumin). Metabolism by the liver produces at least 2 active metabolites which also have antioestrogenic activity. Elimination predominantly via faeces with <10% administered dose excreted in the urine. The elimination half-life is approximately 5–6 days.

Trastuzumab

Herceptin® (POM)

- 150mg powder for concentrate for solution for infusion.

Indications

- Metastatic or early breast cancer or gastro-oesophageal cancer where tumours have either HER2 overexpression or HER2 gene amplification as determined by a validated assay.

Contraindications and precautions

- Trastuzumab is contraindicated in patients with severe dyspnoea at rest.
- Caution should be exercised in patients with pre-existing symptomatic heart failure, hypertension, or documented coronary artery disease.
- All candidates for treatment with trastuzumab should undergo baseline cardiac assessment including history and physical examination, ECG, echocardiogram, or MUGA (multigated acquisition) scan or magnetic resonance imaging.
- Cardiac function should be monitored during treatment (e.g. every 12 weeks) to help identify patients who develop cardiac dysfunction. Patients with early breast cancer should have additional assessments 6-monthly until 24 months after their last administered trastuzumab. Yearly monitoring after an anthracycline is recommended.
- Anthracyclines should be avoided for up to 25 weeks after stopping trastuzumab, as the drug may persist in the circulation. Trastuzumab and anthracyclines should not be given concurrently other than in the neoadjuvant treatment of breast cancer or as part of a clinical study.

☺ Undesirable effects

Very common

- Abdominal pain
- Arthralgia
- Asthenia
- Changes in blood pressure
- Conjunctivitis
- Cough
- Decrease in LVEF
- Diarrhoea
- Dizziness
- Dyspnoea
- Epistaxis
- Facial swelling
- Febrile neutropenia
- Fevers
- Headache
- Hot flushes
- Influenza-like symptoms
- ↑ lacrimation
- Myalgia
- Nausea
- Palpitations
- Rash
- Rhinorrhoea
- Tremor
- Vomiting
- Wheeze.

Common

- Alopecia
- Anorexia
- Anxiety
- Arrhythmias
- Asthma
- Cardiomyopathy
- Confusion
- Constipation
- Depression
- Dry eyes
- Dry mouth
- Dyspepsia

- Haemorrhoids
- Hypersensitivity
- Infections
- Insomnia
- Liver dysfunction
- Mastitis
- Musculoskeletal pain

- Myelosuppression
- Pancreatitis
- Peripheral neuropathy
- Peripheral oedema
- Skin and nail disorders
- Weight change.

Uncommon
- Deafness

- Sepsis.

Rare
- Jaundice

- Pneumonitis.

Not known
- Anaphylaxis
- Cerebral oedema
- Hepatic failure
- Hyperkalaemia
- Hypoprothrombinaemia
- Lung infiltrates
- Oligohydramnios

- Papilloedema
- Pericardial effusion
- Pericarditis
- Pulmonary fibrosis
- Pulmonary oedema
- Respiratory failure
- Retinal haemorrhage.

Drug interactions
- No pharmacokinetic interactions are described.
- Taxanes, gemcitabine, vinorelbine, and radiation therapy may increase the risk of pulmonary toxicity.

Dose
- A loading dose is administered as a 90min IV infusion. If the initial dose was well tolerated, subsequent doses can be administered as a 30min infusion.
- Loading dose of 8mg/kg, followed by 6mg/kg at 3-weekly intervals *or* (breast cancer only) a loading dose of 4mg/kg, followed by 2mg/kg every week.
- Patients with metastatic breast cancer or metastatic gastric cancer should be treated with trastuzumab until progression of disease. Patients with early breast cancer should be treated with trastuzumab for 1 year or until disease recurrence, whichever occurs first.

Dose adjustments
Dose reduction
- Patients may continue trastuzumab therapy at full dose during periods of reversible, chemotherapy-induced myelosuppression.

Cardiac dysfunction
- If the LVEF drops 10 points from baseline *and* to below 50%, treatment should be suspended.

Pharmacology
Trastuzumab is a recombinant humanized IgG1 monoclonal antibody against HER2. As a result, trastuzumab inhibits the proliferation of human tumour cells that overexpress HER2. Additionally, trastuzumab is a potent mediator of ADCC.

Treosulfan

Ovastat® (POM)
- Capsules for oral administration: 250mg.
- Powder for solution for injection or infusion: 1g, 5g.

Indications
- Relapsed ovarian cancer
- Malignancy refractory to standard therapy
- ¥ Ocular melanoma.

Contraindications
- History of hypersensitivity to treosulfan
- Severe bone marrow suppression.

Precautions
- Risk of mucositis: advise patients to swallow capsules whole.
- Risk of haemorrhagic cystitis: advise patients to ↑ fluid intake during therapy.
- ❶ Vesicant: tissue damage if extravasation.
- Fertility:
  - Advise barrier contraception during and for 3 months after therapy.
  - Risk of sterility—advise sperm storage for men.

☺ Undesirable effects
Common
- Alopecia (generally mild)
- Bronze skin discoloration (reversible)
- Myelosuppression (nadir 28 days after therapy)—dose-limiting toxicity
- Nausea and vomiting.

Uncommon
- Secondary malignancies.

Rare
- Addison's disease
- Haemorrhagic cystitis.

Drug interactions
- NSAIDs: ↓ efficacy reported (case report).

🔧 Dose
Monotherapy
- 3 alternative regimens (note all result in total dose of 21–28g during the first 8 weeks of therapy):
  - Regimen A: 1g daily, given in 4 divided doses for 4 weeks, followed by 4 weeks off therapy.
  - Regimen B: 1g daily given in 4 divided doses for 2 weeks, followed by 2 weeks off therapy.
  - Regimen C: 1.5g daily, given in 3 divided doses for 1 week, followed by 3 weeks off therapy. If no evidence of haematological toxicity increase to 2g daily in 4 divided doses for 1 week for subsequent cycles.

..∫ **Dose adjustments**

- If WBC <3.0 × 10^6 or platelets <100 × 10^6 treatment should be interrupted and restarted after 1–2 weeks when haematological parameters are satisfactory with the following dose modifications:
  - Regimen A/B: daily dose reduced to 750mg (500mg if required).
  - Regimen C: daily dose reduced to 1.5g (1g if required).

Renal impairment

- Caution should be exercised as renally excreted.

⊹ **Pharmacology**

Treosulfan is an alkylating agent that mediates cytotoxicity through inter-action of reactive epoxide metabolites with DNA. Treosulfan is well absorbed orally (97%) with maximum concentration 90min after oral dosing. Excretion is renal, with an elimination half-life of 2 hours.

Triptorelin

Decapeptyl® SR (POM)
- Powder for suspension for injection: 3mg, 11.25mg, or 22.5mg.

Indications
- Hormone-dependent locally advanced and metastatic prostate cancer.
- As adjuvant treatment following radiotherapy in patients with high-risk localized or locally advanced prostate cancer.

Contraindications and precautions
- Contraindicated in patients who have already undergone surgical castration (triptorelin will not further decrease testosterone levels).
- Contraindicated as monotherapy in patients with spinal metastases or spinal cord compression due to risk of tumour flare.
- Should be used with caution in patients with ↑ risk of osteoporosis.

☺ Undesirable effects

Common
- Bone demineralization (proportional to time on treatment)
- Fatigue
- Hot flushes
- Nausea/diarrhoea
- Paraesthesia
- Reduced libido
- Weight gain.

Uncommon
- Alopecia
- Altered taste/sense of smell
- Arthralgia/myalgia
- Depression
- Gout
- Gynaecomastia/breast tenderness
- Headache
- Hypertension
- Tinnitus.

Rare
- Changes in glucose tolerance
- Dry mouth
- Flatulence
- Hepatic dysfunction
- Nasopharyngitis
- Pituitary apoplexy
- Thrombocytopenia/leucopenia
- Vertigo
- Visual disturbance.

Drug interactions

Pharmacokinetic
- No specific pharmacokinetic interactions have been reported.

Pharmacodynamic
- Drugs which raise prolactin levels should not be used concomitantly as they can reduce the level of GnRH receptors in the pituitary.

♟ Dose
- 3mg injection IM every month.
- 11.25mg injection IM every 3 months.
- 22.5mg injection IM every 6 months.

Dose adjustments
- To continue on treatment as long as patient is tolerating and disease is under control.

Additional information
- Testosterone levels can initially rise during first 3–4 days on treatment.
- Antiandrogen cover starting 3 days prior to triptorelin therapy and continuing for first 2–3 weeks of treatment can prevent initial tumour flare.

Pharmacology

Triptorelin is a decapeptide analogue of GnRH. Triptorelin treatment initially increases circulating levels of LH and FSH, leading to a transient rise in testosterone. Continuing treatment with triptorelin inhibits LH/FSH secretion and so ↓ testosterone production, usually after 2–3 weeks of therapy.

Vemurafenib

Zelboraf® (POM)
- Tablets: 240mg.

Indications
- Adult patients with BRAF V600 mutation-positive unresectable or metastatic melanoma.

Contraindications and precautions
- Vemurafenib can cause cutaneous squamous cell carcinomas (cuSCCs):
  - All patients should have a full skin examination prior to starting vemurafenib and be monitored routinely while on therapy and up to 6 months after cessation of drug.
  - Any suspicious skin lesions should be excised, sent for dermatopathological evaluation and treated as per local standard of care.
- Vemurafenib can cause QT prolongation:
  - Treatment with vemurafenib is not recommended in patients with uncorrectable electrolyte abnormalities, long QT syndrome, or who are taking other drugs known to prolong the QT interval.
  - ECGs and electrolytes (including Mg) must be monitored in all patients at baseline, after 1 month of treatment, and after dose modification.
- Vemurafenib can cause significant photosensitivity. Patients on vemurafenib should avoid sun exposure, wear protective clothing, and use a broad spectrum (UVA & UVB) sunscreen and lip balm of ≥SPF 30.

☺ Undesirable effects
Common
- Arthralgia/myalgia
- Cough
- Diarrhoea
- Fatigue
- Keratoacanthomas/cuSCC

- Nausea/vomiting/anorexia
- Peripheral oedema
- Photosensitivity reaction
- Pyrexia.

Uncommon
- Basal cell carcinomas
- PPE
- Transaminitis/hyperbilirubinaemia
- Uveitis.

Rare
- Peripheral neuropathy
- Retinal vein occlusion
- Stevens–Johnson syndrome/toxic epidermal necrolysis
- Vasculitis.

Drug interactions

Pharmacokinetic

- Vemurafenib induces CYP3A4 and inhibits CYP1A2, so may:
  - ↓ plasma exposure of drugs metabolized by CYP3A4 (including oral contraceptives)
  - ↑ plasma exposure of drugs metabolized by CYP1A2
  - ↑ warfarin exposure.
- Vemurafenib is metabolized by CYP3A4 and therefore should be used with caution in combination with potent inhibitors of CYP3A4.
- Vemurafenib is a substrate of the efflux transporter P-gp and therefore concomitant treatment with potent P-gp inducers should be avoided.

Pharmacodynamic

- There is evidence that BRAF inhibitors like vemurafenib have ↑ efficacy and ↓ incidence of cuSCC when combined with MEK inhibitors. This is currently being investigated further in clinical trials.

♣ Dose

- 960mg PO BD.

♣ Dose adjustments

- For grade 3 or intolerable grade 2 toxicity, interrupt treatment until toxicity is reduced to grade 0 or 1, then resume at 720mg BD. If similar toxicity recurs, dose reduce further to 480mg BD.
- For grade 4 toxicity, either discontinue or interrupt treatment until toxicity is reduced to grade 0 or 1, then resume at 480mg BD. If similar toxicity recurs, discontinue treatment.
- Dose reductions below 480mg BD are not recommended.
- If the patient develops cuSCC, treatment should be continued without dose adjustment.

Additional information

- Tablets should be swallowed whole with water and not crushed or chewed.

♦ Pharmacology

Vemurafenib is an orally available inhibitor of BRAF, a serine threonine kinase in the MAP kinase cell signalling pathway. It is rapidly absorbed with a median T_{max} of about 4 hours. Mutations in the *BRAF* gene lead to constitutively activated BRAF proteins, which drive cell proliferation and survival in many cancers. Vemurafenib inhibits V600 mutated BRAF kinases, thus reducing downstream ERK phosphorylation and cellular proliferation. Vemurafenib is primarily metabolized in the liver by the CYP3A4 enzyme and excreted in bile and faeces.

Vinblastine

Vinblastine sulphate, Velban® (POM)
- Solution for injection: 1mg/1ml, 10mg/10ml.

Indications
- Advanced testicular cancer
- Breast carcinoma
- Hodgkin and non-Hodgkin lymphoma
- Kaposi's sarcoma.

Contraindications
- ❶ For IV administration only —fatal if given by other routes.
- Hypersensitivity to vinblastine.

Precautions
- ❶ Highly vesicant: severe tissue damage associated with extravasation.
- Choose largest vein in an extremity free from circulatory compromise for administration.
- Avoid exposure during pregnancy.
- Liver dysfunction: use with caution due to ↑↑ risk of neuropathy.
- Fertility:
  - Advise barrier contraception during and for 3 months after therapy.
  - Risk of sterility—advise sperm storage for men.

NB Manufacturer recommends subcutaneous injection of hyaluronidase and application of heat to help disperse drug in cases of extravasation.

☺ Undesirable effects
Common
- Myelosuppression (leucopenia)—dose-limiting toxicity
- Neurotoxicity (dose-dependent):
  - Autonomic neuropathy
  - Peripheral neuropathy
  - Raynaud's phenomenon.

Uncommon
- Alopecia
- Bronchospasm/dyspnoea
- Nausea and vomiting (minimal emetic risk).

Rare
- Abdominal pain/diarrhoea
- Jaw pain
- Pulmonary oedema
- SIADH.

Drug interactions
- Taxanes: ↑ risk of neurotoxicity.
- Cytochrome P450 inhibitors: may ↓ vinblastine metabolism resulting in ↑ toxicity.

- Phenytoin: vinblastine may ↓ levels.
- Mitomycin: avoid combination due to ↑ risk of pulmonary toxicity.

Dose

Combination therapy
- 6–10mg/m^2 every 2–4 weeks in combination.

Other
- 4–10mg/m^2 weekly as monotherapy.
- As a continuous infusion dosed at 1.7–2mg/m^2/24 hours over a 96-hour period.

Dose adjustments

Myelosuppression
- SPC advises dose escalation depending on nadir leucocyte count.

Hepatic impairment
- Consider dose reduction for hepatic insufficiency due to ↑ risk of neurotoxicity.

Pharmacology

Vinblastine is a plant alkaloid that binds to microtubules, resulting in inhibition of mitotic spindle formation and metaphase arrest. Vinblastine-induced cytotoxicity may also result from effects on nucleic acid and protein synthesis. Vinblastine is poorly absorbed by mouth. Following IV administration, vinblastine is rapidly distributed throughout most tissues, though CSF penetration is poor. Vinblastine is metabolized in the liver by CYP3A to its active metabolite 4-deacetylvinblastine and eliminated via the hepatobiliary route. ~14% vinblastine is eliminated in the urine. The half-life is 20–24 hours.

Vincristine

Oncovin®

- Non-proprietary formulation also available.
- 1mg/ml concentrate for IV infusion.

Indications

- Leukaemia: AML, ALL, CLL, and CML in blast crisis
- Hodgkin and non-Hodgkin lymphoma
- Multiple myeloma (rarely used)
- Solid tumours including breast, bronchogenic, head and neck and soft tissue sarcoma
- Paediatric solid tumours, e.g. neuroblastoma, Wilms' tumour, Ewing's sarcoma.

Contraindications and precautions

- ❶Only use intravenously—*fatal if given intrathecally*.
- Caution in elderly or those with pre-existing neuropathy.
- Ensure good IV access as can cause ulceration if extravasates.

☺ Undesirable effects

Common

- Alopecia.
- Constipation
- ❶ Fatal if given intrathecally
- Myelosuppression is *not* a common side effect with single agent vincristine
- Neuropathy – elderly or those with pre-existing neuropathy are more at risk
- Rash.

Uncommon

- Nausea
- Paralytic ileus
- SIADH
- Vomiting.

Rare

- Acute shortness of breath and severe bronchospasm.

Drug interactions

Pharmacokinetic

- When used in combination with L-asparaginase, should administer vincristine 12–24 hours before the drug (L-asparaginase may reduce hepatic clearance of vincristine and increase toxicity).

Pharmacodynamic

- Myelosuppressive effect potentiated by allopurinol, isoniazid, pyrazinamide (mechanism unclear).
- Pulmonary complications appear particularly to occur when vincristine used in combination with mitomycin.

♪ Dose
● 1.4–1.5mg/m^2 in adults, usually with a cap at 2mg.

♪ Dose adjustments
● Reduce dose in hepatic impairment: 50% reduction when bilirubin >51micromol/L.

♦ Pharmacology
Vincristine binds to tubulin dimers inhibiting assembly of microtubular structures. This arrests mitosis in metaphase due to interruption of spindle formation.

Vindesine

Eldisine® (POM)

- Powder for solution for injection: 5mg.

Indications

- Hodgkin and non-Hodgkin lymphoma
- Acute leukaemia.

Contraindications

- ❶ For IV administration only—*fatal if given by other routes.*
- Demyelinating form of Charcot–Marie–Tooth syndrome.
- Hypersensitivity to vindesine.

Precautions

- ❶ Highly vesicant: severe tissue damage associated with extravasation.
- Choose largest vein in an extremity free from circulatory compromise for administration.
- Liver dysfunction: use with caution due to ↑↑ risk of neuropathy.
- Fertility:
  - Advise barrier contraception during and for 3 months after therapy.
  - Risk of sterility—advise sperm storage for men.

NB Manufacturer recommends subcutaneous injection of hyaluronidase and application of heat to help disperse drug in cases of extravasation.

☺ Undesirable effects

Common

- Myelosuppression (granulocytopenia)—dose-limiting toxicity
- Neurotoxicity (dose-dependent):
  - Autonomic neuropathy
  - Peripheral neuropathy
  - Raynaud's phenomenon.

Uncommon

- Alopecia
- Bronchospasm/dyspnoea
- Nausea and vomiting (minimal emetic risk).

Rare

- Abdominal pain/diarrhoea
- Jaw pain
- Pulmonary oedema
- SIADH.

Drug interactions

- Taxanes: ↑ risk of neurotoxicity
- Cytochrome P450 inhibitors: may ↓ vindesine metabolism resulting in ↑ toxicity
- Phenytoin: vindesine may ↓ levels
- Mitomycin: avoid combination due to ↑ risk of pulmonary toxicity.

Dose

Combination therapy

- 3mg/m^2 weekly to increase to 4mg/m^2 in 0.5mg/m^2 depending on myelosuppression.

Dose adjustments

Myelosuppression

- SPC advises dose escalation depending on nadir leucocyte count.

Hepatic impairment

- Consider dose reduction for hepatic insufficiency due to ↑ risk of neurotoxicity.

Pharmacology

Vindesine is a plant alkaloid with similar mechanism of action, metabolism and excretion to vinblastine.

Vinorelbine

Navelbine® (POM)
- 10mg/ml concentrate for solution for infusion.
- 20mg, 30mg, and 80mg soft capsules.

Indications
- First-line treatment of stage 3 or 4 NSCLC.
- Advanced breast cancer stage 3 and 4 relapsing after or refractory to an anthracycline-containing regimen.

Contraindications and precautions
- Vinorelbine is contraindicated in GI disease significantly affecting absorption.
- Avoid in severe hepatic insufficiency and in those on long-term oxygen therapy.
- Avoid live attenuated vaccines.
- Vinorelbine should not be given concomitantly with radiotherapy if the treatment field includes the liver.
- Use with caution in patients with ischaemic heart disease.
- Due to sorbitol content, patients with rare hereditary problems with fructose intolerance should not take the capsules.

☺ Undesirable effects

Very common
- Abdominal pain
- Alopecia
- Anorexia
- Bacterial, viral, or fungal infections without neutropenia
- Constipation
- Diarrhoea
- Fatigue
- Fever
- Gastric disorders
- Myelosuppression
- Nausea
- Neurosensory disorders, generally limited to loss of tendon reflexes and infrequently severe
- Skin reactions
- Stomatitis
- Vomiting
- Weight loss.

Common
- Arthralgia including jaw pain
- Bacterial, viral or fungal infections resulting from bone marrow depression
- Chills
- Cough
- Dizziness
- Dysphagia
- Dyspnoea
- Dysuria and other genitourinary disorder
- Febrile neutropenia
- Headache
- Hepatic disorders
- Hypertension
- Hypotension
- Insomnia
- Myalgia
- Neuromotor disorders
- Neutropenic infection
- Oesophagitis
- Pain including pain at the tumour site
- Taste disorders
- Visual disorders
- Weight gain.

Uncommon
- Ataxia
- Paralytic ileus (rarely fatal), treatment may be resumed after recovery of normal bowel mobility.

Not known
- GI bleeding.
- Myocardial infarction in patients with cardiac medical history or cardiac risk factors
- Neutropenic sepsis
- Severe hyponatraemia.

☺ Undesirable effects associated with IV use only
Uncommon
- Bronchospasm.
- Flushing and peripheral coldness
- Septicaemia (very rarely fatal)

Rare
- Interstitial pneumonitis
- Pancreatitis.
- Severe hypotension

Not known
- SIADH
- Systemic allergic reactions were reported as anaphylaxis, anaphylactic shock or anaphylactoid type reaction.

Drug interactions
Pharmacokinetic
- CYP3A4 is involved in the metabolism of vinorelbine, so combination with strong inhibitors of the isoenzyme can increase blood concentrations of vinorelbine and combination with strong inducers of this isoenzyme decrease blood concentrations.

⚗ Dose
Monotherapy (IV administration)
- 25–30mg/m^2 infusion once weekly.

Combination regimen (IV administration)
- 25–30mg/m^2 infusion, with reduced frequency of administration, e.g. day 1 and day 5 every 3 weeks or day 1 and day 8 every 3 weeks, according to treatment protocol.

Monotherapy (oral administration)
- 60mg/m^2 once weekly, for the first 3 administrations. Beyond the 3rd administration, it is recommended to increase the dose of vinorelbine to 80mg/m^2 once weekly if blood counts permit.

Combination regimen (oral administration)
- For combination regimens, the dose and schedule will be adapted to the treatment protocol. Based on clinical studies, the oral dose of 80mg/m^2 was demonstrated to correspond to 30mg/m^2 of the IV form and 60mg/m^2 to 25mg/m^2.

Other
- Even for patients with BSA $\geq 2m^2$ the total dose should never exceed 120mg per week at $60mg/m^2$ and 160mg per week at $80mg/m^2$.
- Intrathecal administration of vinorelbine may be fatal.

Dose adjustments
- In patients with moderate liver impairment (bilirubin from 1.5–3 × ULN), vinorelbine should be administered at a dose of $50mg/m^2$/week (orally) or $20mg/m^2$ (intravenously).
- No dose alteration required for impaired renal function.
- Dose reductions of 20–50% should be considered for patients experiencing grade 3–4 haematological or non- haematological toxicities.

Pharmacology
- Vinorelbine is a vinca alkaloid and acts on the dynamic equilibrium of tubulin in the microtubular apparatus of the cell. Vinorelbine blocks mitosis at G2–M, causing cell death in interphase or at the following mitosis.

Index